O G P L
OXFORD GENERAL PRACTICE LIBRARY

Cancer Care

O G P L

OXFORD GENERAL PRACTICE LIBRARY

Cancer Care

Max Watson

Lecturer, Palliative Medicine,
University of Ulster,
Honorary Consultant Palliative Medicine,
Northern Ireland Hospice,
Belfast, and Princess Alice Hospice,
Esher, and Clinical Adviser,
Hospice Friendly Hospitals Program,
Dublin

Chantal Simon

General Practitioner, Bournemouth,
Dorset, and Editor of InnovAiT

and Series Editor

Audrey Fenton

Specialist Registrar Medical Oncology,
Belfast City Hospital

Anne Drake

Consultant in Clinical Oncology,
Belfast City Hospital

Caroline McLoughlin

Consultant in Palliative Medicine,
Northern Trust, Coleraine

Richard Wilson

Consultant/Senior Lecturer in Oncology,
Clinical Director, N. Ireland Cancer Clinical Trials Unit
Centre for Cancer Research and Cell Biology,
Queen's University,
Belfast Cancer Centre, Belfast

OXFORD

UNIVERSITY PRESS

OXFORD
UNIVERSITY PRESS

Great Clarendon Street, Oxford OX2 6DP

Oxford University Press is a department of the University of Oxford.
It furthers the University's objective of excellence in research, scholarship,
and education by publishing worldwide in

Oxford New York

Auckland Cape Town Dar es Salaam Hong Kong Karachi
Kuala Lumpur Madrid Melbourne Mexico City Nairobi
New Delhi Shanghai Taipei Toronto

With offices in

Argentina Austria Brazil Chile Czech Republic France Greece
Guatemala Hungary Italy Japan Poland Portugal Singapore
South Korea Switzerland Thailand Turkey Ukraine Vietnam

Oxford is a registered trade mark of Oxford University Press
in the UK and in certain other countries

Published in the United States
by Oxford University Press Inc., New York

© Oxford University Press, 2010

The moral rights of the authors have been asserted
Database right Oxford University Press (maker)

First published 2010

British Library Cataloguing in Publication Data

Data available

Library of Congress Cataloging in Publication Data

Data available

Typeset by Newgen Imaging Systems (P) Ltd., Chennai, India
Printed in Great Britain
on acid-free paper by
Ashford Colour Press Ltd., Gosport, Hampshire

ISBN 978–0–19–923203–1

10 9 8 7 6 5 4 3 2 1

Whilst every effort has been made to ensure that the contents of this book are as
complete, accurate and up-to-date as possible at the date of writing. Oxford
University Press is not able to give any guarantee or assurance that such is the case.
Readers are urged to take appropriately qualified medical advice in all cases. The
information in this book is intended to be useful to the general reader, but should
not be used as a means o self-diagnosis or for the prescription of medication.

Contents

Symbols and abbreviations *vii*

Symbols and abbreviations

α FP	Alpha-fetoprotein
AA	Attendance Allowance
ACE	Angiotensin-converting enzyme
ACTH	Adenocorticotropic hormone
ADH	Antidiuretic hormone
AF	Atrial fibrillation
AIDS	Acquired immunodeficiency syndrome
ALL	Acute lymphoblastic leukaemia
AML	Acute myeloid leukaemia
BCC	Basal cell carcinoma
BCG	Bacille Calmette-Guérin
BD	Twice daily
BM	Finger-prick capillary blood glucose
BMA	British Medical Association
BP	Blood pressure
BSO	Bilateral salpingo-oophorectomy
ᶜ	Cochrane review
CEA	Carcinoembryonic antigen
CF	Correction factor
cGIN	Cervical glandular intraepithelial neoplasia
CHD	Congestive heart disease
CHOP	Cyclophosphamide, hydroxydaunorubicin (Adriamycin), Oncovin (vincristine), and prednisone/prednisolone
CIN	Cutaneous intraepithelial neoplasia
CLL	Chronic lymphocytic leukaemia
CML	Chronic myeloid leukaemia
CNS	Central nervous system
COC	Combined oral contraceptive
COPD	Chronic obstructive pulmonary disease
CPR	Cardiopulmonary resuscitation
Cr	Creatinine
CRP	C-reactive protein
CT	Computed tomography

CVAD	Central venous access device
CXR	Chest X-ray
dl	Decilitre
DLA	Disability Living Allowance
DLBCL	Diffuse large B cell
DM	Diabetes mellitus
DN	District nurse
DNA	Deoxyribonucleic acid
DRE	Digital rectal examination
DVP	Deep vein thrombosis
DWP	Department of Work and Pensions
e.g.	For example
EBV	Epstein–Barr virus
ECG	Electrocardiogram
ECOG	Eastern Co-operative Oncology Group
eGFR	Estimated glomerular filtration rate
EPA	Enduring power of attorney
ESR	Erythrocyte sedimentation rate
ERCP	Endoscopic retrograde cholangiopancreatography
FBC	Full blood count
FDG	[18F]-fluorodeoxyglucose
FH	Family history
FOB	Faecal occult blood
FU	Fluorouracil
GFR	Growth factor receptor
GI	Gastrointestinal
GIST	Gastrointestinal stromal tumour
GMC	General Medical Council
GMS	General Medical Services
GnRH	Gonadotropin-releasing hormone agonist
GP	General Practitioner
GSA	Global Sum Allocation
GSE	Global Sum Equivalent
h.	Hour
HAART	Highly active anti-retroviral therapy
HCC	Hepatocellular carcinoma
Hb	Haemoglobin
hCG	Human chorionic gonadotropin
HIV	Human immunodeficiency virus

HMMA	4-hydroxy-3-methoxymandelic acid
HPV	Human papilloma virus
HRP	Home Responsibilities Protection
HRT	Hormone replacement therapy
HSV	Herpes simplex virus
IgM	Immunoglobulin M
IM	Intramuscular
INR	International normalized ratio
ITP	Idiopathic thrombocytopenic purpura
IUCD	Intrauterine contraceptive device
IV	Intravenous
LH	Lutenizing hormone
LHRH	Lutenizing hormone releasing hormone
LLETZ	Large loop excision of the transformation zone
LMWH	Low-molecular weight heparin
LN	Lymph node
LSD	D-lysergic acid diethylamide
LVF	Left ventricular failure
MALT	Mucosa-associated lymphoid tissue
mcg	Microgram
MEN	Multiple endocrine neoplasia
mg	Milligram
MGUS	Monoclonal gammopathy of uncertain significance
MHRA	Medicines and Healthcare Products Regulatory Agency
MI	Myocardial infarction
mm	Millimetre
mmol	Millimol
MND	Motor neurone disease
mo	Month
MPIG	Minimum practice income guarantee
MRI	Magnetic resonance imaging
MST	Morphine sulphate tablet
MSU	Mid-stream specimen of urine
NHL	Non-Hodgkin lymphoma
NI	National Insurance
NSAID	Non-steroidal anti-inflammatory drug
od	Once daily
OT	Occupational therapist
PCO	Primary care organization

PE	Pulmonary embolus
PET	Positron emission tomography
PICC	Peripherally inserted central catheter
PiL	Patient information leaflet
PLAP	Placental alkaline phosphatase
PMB	Post menopausal bleed
PMH	Past medical history
PO	Per oral
PPI	Proton pump inhibitor
PPP	Primary proliferative polycythaemia
PR	Per rectum
prn	As needed
PS	Performance status
PSA	Prostate specific antigen
R	Randomized controlled trial in major journal
RBC	Red blood cell
S	Systemic review in major journal
SC	subcutaneous
TAH	Total abdominal hysterectomy
TCC	Transitional cell carcinoma
tds	Three times a day
TFTs	Thyroid function tests
TNM	Tumour, node, metastasis
TTS	Transdermal therapeutic
TURBT	Transurethral resection of the bladder tumour
U&E	Urea and electrolytes
UC	Ulcerative colitis
UK	United Kingdom
UMN	Upper motor neurone
US	United States
USS	Ultrasound scan
UTI	Urinary tract infection
VIN	Venous intraepithelial neoplasia
VMA	Vanillylmandelic acid
VQ	Ventilation-perfusion
WCC	White cell count
WHO	World Health Organization
wk	Week
y	Year

Chapter 1

Cancer in the UK

1

Incidence of cancer in the UK

In most industrialized countries cancer is a major cause of morbidity and mortality. In the United Kingdom (UK), where cancer has overtaken heart disease as the leading cause of death:
- One person in three will be diagnosed with cancer during their lifetime
- One person in four will die from cancer.

Each year in the UK:
- A quarter of a million people are diagnosed with cancer
- Approximately 120,000 people die from cancer
- The average GP will see eight or nine patients with new cancer diagnoses.

Incidence in adults: Approximately 60% of all cancers are diagnosed in those aged over 65y. As we live in an ageing population, the impact of cancer is increasing. Although there are >200 different types of cancer, breast, lung, large bowel (colorectal), prostate, and skin cancer account for over 50% of all new cases. See Figure 1.1 and Table 1.1.

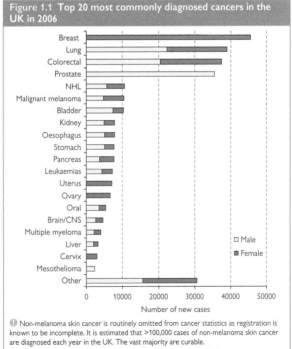

Figure 1.1 **Top 20 most commonly diagnosed cancers in the UK in 2006**

Number of new cases

ⓘ Non-melanoma skin cancer is routinely omitted from cancer statistics as registration is known to be incomplete. It is estimated that >100,000 cases of non-melanoma skin cancer are diagnosed each year in the UK. The vast majority are curable.

Statistics in Figure 1.1 are reproduced with permission from Cancer Research UK.

Table 1.1 Risk of being diagnosed with cancer over a lifetime

Site	% of cohort that develop cancer over lifetime*		Lifetime risk	
	Male	Female	Male	Female
Bladder	3.3 (0.7)	1.3 (0.2)	1 in 30	1 in 79
Brain and CNS	0.7 (0.4)	0.5 (0.3)	1 in 147	1 in 207
Breast	1 in 100	10.9 (5.6)	≈1 in 900	1 in 9
Cervix	–	0.9 (0.6)	–	1 in 116
Kidney	1.1 (0.4)	0.6 (0.2)	1 in 89	1 in 162
Large bowel	5.7 (1.4)	4.9 (1.1)	1 in 18	1 in 20
Leukaemia	1.0 (0.4)	0.8 (0.3)	1 in 95	1 in 127
Lung	8.0 (1.7)	4.3 (1.0)	1 in 13	1 in 23
Melanoma	0.7 (0.4)	0.9 (0.5)	1 in 147	1 in 117
Multiple myeloma	0.6 (0.1)	0.5 (0.1)	1 in 177	1 in 204
Non-Hodgkin lymphoma	1.4 (0.6)	1.2 (0.4)	1 in 69	1 in 83
Oesophagus	1.3 (0.4)	1.1 (0.2)	1 in 75	1 in 95
Ovary	–	2.1 (0.9)	–	1 in 48
Pancreas	1.0 (0.3)	1.1 (0.2)	1 in 96	1 in 95
Prostate	7.3 (0.9)	–	1 in 14	–
Stomach	2.3 (0.5)	1.2 (0.2)	1 in 44	1 in 86
Uterus	–	1.4 (0.6)	–	1 in 73

* % in brackets is that developing cancer by age 65y.

Statistics in Table 1.1 are reproduced with permission from Cancer Research UK.

Incidence in children: Many types of cancer that occur in children are only rarely seen in adults. Conversely, most cancers commonly seen in adults are rarely seen in children. Approximately 1,500 new cases of childhood cancer are diagnosed each year in the UK, 20% more in boys than in girls. Risk of being diagnosed with childhood cancer (i.e. cancer in an individual of <15y of age) is:
- Overall 1 in 500
- Overall 1 in 1,600 for leukaemia
- Overall 1 in 2,200 for a brain/spinal tumour
- Overall 1 in 1,100 for all other cancers combined.

Cancer mortality

In 2005 in the UK, there were 153,491 deaths from cancer—one in four of all deaths (29% ♂; 24% ♀). Lung cancer is the most common cause of cancer death in both men and women (Figures 1.2 and 1.3). Cigarette smoking has been identified as the most important cause of preventable death in the UK, with one in three deaths from cancer and 88% of all lung cancer deaths being linked to smoking.

Childhood cancer deaths: There are approximately 300 deaths/year in the UK from cancer amongst children aged <15y—33% more in boys than girls. This accounts for a quarter of the deaths of children aged 5–14y and 15% of deaths of children aged 1–4y. Leukaemias (32%) and brain/spinal tumours (30%) are the most common causes of cancer deaths amongst children.

Age of death: 76% of deaths from cancer occur in people aged >65y. Death rates rise with increasing age. However, cancer causes a greater proportion of deaths in younger people and is responsible for 37% of deaths in those <65y (47% of deaths in women; 31% in men).

Trends in mortality: Overall, mortality from cancer decreased by 17% (from 218 to 180/100,000 population) in the 30y up to 2005, despite increasing incidence of cancer over that same time period (Figure 1.4). Male mortality is higher than female mortality but decreasing at a faster rate.

4

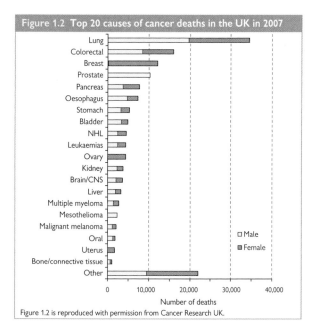

Figure 1.2 **Top 20 causes of cancer deaths in the UK in 2007**

Number of deaths

Figure 1.2 is reproduced with permission from Cancer Research UK.

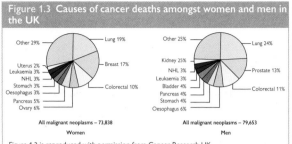

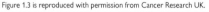

Figure 1.3 Causes of cancer deaths amongst women and men in the UK

Figure 1.3 is reproduced with permission from Cancer Research UK.

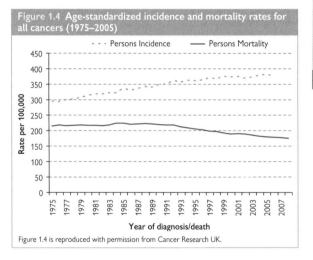

Figure 1.4 Age-standardized incidence and mortality rates for all cancers (1975–2005)

Figure 1.4 is reproduced with permission from Cancer Research UK.

Cancer survival

Cancers are grouped into three survival bands:
- ≥50%
- 10%–49%, and
- <10%.

Five-year relative survival rates are increasing for most cancers and the overall 5y survival rate has now reached 50%. The 5y survival rate in women (56%) is higher than that in men (43%) and this gender gap is also seen for 10y survival rates (39% vs. 52%).

49% of cancers diagnosed in women and 30% of cancers diagnosed in men fall into the highest survival category (Figure 1.5). The highest 5y survival rate for men is for testicular cancer (96%) and that for women is for malignant melanoma (87%).

Age, deprivation, and survival: Among adults, relative survival goes down with increasing age at diagnosis for almost all cancers, even when higher mortality from other causes in older age groups is allowed for. Cancer survival for adults is generally lower for more deprived patients, even when higher all-cause mortality is allowed for.

Childhood cancer survival: 75% of children with cancer in the UK survive 5y. After surviving for 5y, 90% of children who have survived cancer can be considered cured. The best survival rates are with retino-blastoma, gonadal germ cell tumours and Hodgkin's lymphoma which have 5y survival rates of ≈95%.

Effect of treatment centre:
- Surgeons treating large numbers of patients tend to produce better results than those treating fewer patients
- Children with cancer do better when treated in specialist centres
- Patients with particular cancers—breast, ovary, oesophagus, pancreas, stomach, testis, and lung—appear to survive longer when treated at specialist centres
- Patients who are in clinical trials may do better.

These observations have influenced the delivery of cancer care throughout the UK (Calman–Hine recommendations). Care is provided through a combination of regional cancer centres and more localized cancer units.

Regional cancer centres: Serve populations ≥ 1 million and treat all cancers. They provide:
- Sophisticated diagnostic imaging: MRI, PET, CT etc.
- Specialist surgical services
- Specialist oncologist services
- Specialist clinical nurse skills: intravenous chemotherapy, palliative care, rehabilitation, psychological support, stoma care, and lymphoedema management
- Radiotherapy services
- Specialist palliative care services
- Multidisciplinary team working: physiotherapy, dietetics, speech therapy, occupational therapy, and social services.

Cancer units: These are based at district/area hospital level and treat common cancers. They have no radiotherapy services but do provide:

- Surgical subspecialization
- Medical subspecialization and delivery of chemotherapy
- Nurse specialists
- Specialist palliative care
- Multidisciplinary team working: physiotherapy, dietetics, speech therapy, occupational therapy, and social services.

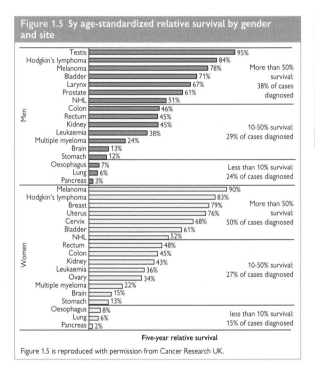

Figure 1.5 **5y age-standardized relative survival by gender and site**

Five-year relative survival

Figure 1.5 is reproduced with permission from Cancer Research UK.

The GP contract and cancer care

The General Medical Services (GMS) Contract: Although there may be some differences in process in each of the four countries of the UK, the principles of the GMS contract apply to all. A total sum for GMS services is given to each primary care organization (PCO) as part of a bigger unified budget allocation. PCOs are responsible for managing the GMS budget locally (Table 1.2).

The contract: A contract is made between an individual practice and a PCO. All the partners of the practice, at least one of whom must be a GP, have to sign the contract. It includes the following:
- National terms applicable to all practices (the 'practice contract')
- Which services will be provided by that practice i.e.
  - Essential
  - Additional—if not opted out
  - Out-of-hours—if not opted out
  - Enhanced—if opted in
- Level of quality of essential and additional services that the practice 'aspires' to
- Support arrangements e.g. information technology (IT), premises
- Total financial resources i.e. global sum + quality achievement payments + enhanced services payments + premises + IT + dispensing.

Essential services: All practices must undertake these services, which include:
- *Day-to-day medical care of the practice population*: health promotion, management of minor and self-limiting illness, and referral to secondary care services and other agencies as appropriate.
- *General management of patients who are terminally ill*
- *Chronic disease management.*

Additional services: Services the practice will usually undertake but may 'opt out' of. If the practice opts out, the PCO takes responsibility for providing the service instead. The practice then receives a ↓ global sum payment.

Enhanced services: Commissioned by the PCO and paid for *in addition* to the global sum payment. These are of three types:
- *Directed Enhanced Services*: services under national direction with national specifications and benchmark pricing which all PCOs must commission to cover their relevant population
- *National Enhanced Services*: services with national minimum standards and benchmark pricing but not directed (i.e. PCOs do not have to provide these services)
- *Services developed locally* to meet local needs (Local Enhanced Services) e.g. enhanced care of the homeless.

Personal Medical Services (PMS) Contracts: These contracts are locally agreed and locally negotiated between practices and PCOs setting out services that will be provided and payment which will be made. PMS contracts do not have to contain all the elements of the GMS contract and can contain additional elements by negotiation.

Table 1.2 Payment under the GMS contract

Payment	Explanation
The global sum	Major part of the money paid to practices. Paid monthly and intended to cover practice running costs. *Includes provision for* • Delivery of essential services and additional/out-of-hours services if not opted out • Staff costs • Career development • Locum reimbursement (e.g. for appraisal, career development, and protected time).
Aspiration payments	Advance payments to allow practices to develop services to achieve higher quality standards. Aspiration payments are made monthly alongside global sum payments and amount to roughly 60% of the points achieved the previous year (for 2010/11 this was ≈2009/10 points achieved × £124.60/point × 60% × list size adjustment).
Achievement payments	Payments made for the practice's achieved number of points in the quality and outcomes framework (📖 p.10) as measured at the start of the following year. Aspiration payments already received are deducted from the total i.e. payment for actual points less aspiration pay.
Payment for 'extra' services	Paid to practices that provide directed enhanced services, national enhanced services, and/or local enhanced services to meet local needs.
MPIG	Protects those practices that lost out under the redistribution effect of the new resource allocation formula. Calculated from the difference between the GSA under the new GMS contract and the GSE—the amount the practice would have earned for providing the same service under the old GMS contract ('The Red Book'). If GSA < GSE a CF will be applied as long as necessary so that GSA + CF = GSE.
Other payments	Payments for premises, IT, and dispensing (dispensing practices only).

ⓘ The Carr-Hill allocation formula is a GMS resource allocation formula for allocating funds for the global sum and quality payments. The formula takes the practice population and then makes a series of adjustments based on the profile of the local community, taking account of determinants of relative practice workload and costs.

The quality and outcomes framework: The quality and outcomes framework (QOF) was developed specifically for the new GMS contract. Financial incentives are used to encourage high-quality care.

The domains: The GMS quality framework is divided into 4 domains,
- Clinical
- Organizational
- Additional services
- Patient experience

See Table 1.3

Indicators: Every domain has a set of 'indicators' which relate to quality standards or guidelines that can be achieved within that domain. The indicators were developed by an expert group based on the best available evidence at the time and are updated regularly. All data should be obtainable from practice clinical systems and Read codes have been developed to make this easier. Indicators are split into three types:
- *Structure* e.g. is a disease register in place?
- *Process*: e.g. is a particular measure being recorded? Is action being taken where appropriate?
- *Outcome*: e.g. how well is the condition being controlled?

Quality points: All achievement against quality indicators converts to points. Each point has a monetary value.
- *Yes/no indicators*: All points are allocated if the result is +ve and none if −ve.
- *Range of attainment*: For most of the clinical indicators it is not possible to attain 100% results (even if allowed exceptions are applied) so a range of satisfactory attainment is specified. Minimum standard is 40%. Points are allocated in a linear fashion based on comparison with attainment against a maximum standard e.g. if the maximum percentage for an indicator is 90%, the minimum 40% and the practice achieves 65%, the practice will receive 25/50 (i.e. half) of the available points.

Annually each practice completes a standard return form recording achievement in the past year. Most practices use the Quality and Outcomes Framework Management and Analysis System (QMAS) to do this. There is also an annual quality review visit by the PCO. Based on achievement, the PCO confirms level of achievement funding attained and discusses points the practice will "aspire" to the following year. The process is confirmed in writing and signed off by both parties. PCO-wide quality is checked against other PCOs countrywide.

The quality framework and the Personal medical services contract: Mechanisms for quality delivery and the quality framework are broadly comparable for GMS and PMS practices. PMS practices have a locally negotiated contract but can apply for aspiration payments and achievement payments in the same way as GMS practices. However, to reflect the local nature of the contracts, standards PMS practices are working towards do not have to be the same as those contained in the National Quality Framework. Nevertheless, all standards must be rigorous, evidence based, monitored fairly, assessed against criteria agreed between PCOs and providers, and paid at appropriate and equitable rates.

Table 1.3 Calculation of points for quality framework payments

Components of total points score:	Points:	Way in which points are calculated:
Clinical indicators	697	Achieving pre-set standards in management of:
		• Asthma • Hypertension
		• Atrial fibrillation • Hypothyroidism
		• Cancer • Learning disability
		• Chronic kidney • Mental health
		disease • Obesity
		• COPD • Stroke and
		• Coronary heart transient
		disease ischaemic attack
		• Dementia • Palliative care
		• Depression • Primary preven-
		• DM tion of cardio-
		• Epilepsy vascular disease
		• Heart failure • Smoking
Organizational	167.5	Achieving pre-set standards in:
		• Records
		• Information for patients
		• Education and training
		• Medicines management
		• Practice management
Additional services	44	Achieving pre-set standards in:
		• Cervical screening
		• Child health surveillance
		• Maternity services
		• Sexual health & contraception
Patient experience	91.5	Achieving pre-set standards in:
		• Patient survey*
		• Consultation length.
Total possible	**1,000**	

In 2009/10 and 2010/11 the average value of 1 point = £124.60

*Both the Improving Practice Questionnaire (IPQ) and General Practice Assessment Questionnaire (GPAQ) are available from CFEP Surveys UK (www.cfepsurveys.co.uk). A charge is payable for usage.

Further information:

NHS Employers ⌨ www.nhsemployers.org
DoH The GMS Contract. ⌨ www.dh.gov.uk
BMA The GMS Contract and supporting documents ⌨ www.bma.org.uk

Cancer and palliative care indicators

Cancer indicators: The cancer indicators (Table 1.4) require the practice to keep a record of patients diagnosed with cancer since 1st April 2003, excluding those diagnosed with non-melanotic skin cancer (Cancer 1). The practice reports the number of patients added to its cancer register in the last 12mo and that number as a proportion of total list size. Verification may involve comparison with expected prevalence data.

Cancer 3 requires practices to ensure that patients' support needs are reviewed within 6mo of diagnosis. Reviews should include the following:
- The individual's health and support needs, *and*
- Co-ordination of care between sectors.

The practice reports the number of patients with cancer diagnosed in the past 18mo with a review recorded <6mo after the practice is informed of diagnosis. Verification may include random selection of case notes to verify that both components of the review have been undertaken and recorded.

Palliative care: 6 points out of a total of 1,000 are available for palliative care (Table 1.4). To achieve these points practices must maintain a register of all patients in need of palliative care/support (palliative care 3) and review all those on the register at a multidisciplinary meeting at least every 3mo (palliative care 2). The practice reports the number of patients on its palliative care register and submits written evidence to the PCO describing the system for initiating and recording review meetings.

Criteria for inclusion on the register are broad. Include patients if:
- Their death in the next 12mo can be reasonably predicted *and/or*
- They have clinical indicators of need for palliative care that are prognostic clinical indicators of advanced or irreversible disease and contain one core and one disease-specific indicator *and/or*
- They are the subject of a DS1500 form (this can be issued if a patient is suffering from a progressive disease and is not expected to survive >6mo).

Core predictors of the need for palliative care are:
- Multiple co-morbidities
- >10% weight loss over 6mo
- General physical decline
- Serum albumin <25g/l
- Reducing performance status/Karnofsky score <50% (Box 1.1)/ dependence in most activities of daily living.

Disease-specific indicator for cancer patients: Any patient whose cancer is metastatic or not amenable to treatment (with some exceptions). This may apply to some cancer patients from diagnosis e.g. lung cancer. The single most important predictive factor in cancer is performance status (Table 4.3, 📖 p.57) and functional ability. If patients are spending >50% of their time in bed/lying down, prognosis is likely to be ≤3mo (Table 1.4).

Table 1.4 Quality and outcomes framework (QOF) indicators for cancer and palliative care

Indicator	Description	Points	Payment stages
Palliative care 3	The practice has a complete register available of all patients in need of palliative care/support irrespective of age.	3	
Palliative care 2	The practice has multi-disciplinary case review meetings at least every 3mo where all patients on the palliative care register are discussed.	3	
Cancer 1	The practice can produce a register of all cancer patients, excluding non-melanotic skin cancer, from 1.4.2003.	5	
Cancer 3	% of patients with cancer, diagnosed <18mo ago who have a patient review recorded as occurring <6mo after the practice received confirmation of diagnosis.	6	40%–90%

Box 1.1 The Karnofsky score. Measures patient performance of activities of daily living

Score (%)	Function
100	Normal, no evidence of disease.
90	Normal activity. Only minor symptoms.
80	Normal activity with effort. Some symptoms.
70	Able to self-care but unable to do normal activities.
60	Requires occasional assistance but cares for most of own needs.
50	Requires considerable assistance.
40	Disabled, requires special assistance.
30	Severely disabled.
20	Very sick, requires active supportive treatment
10	Moribund

Chapter 2

Prevention of cancer

'It is a wise man's part to avoid sickness rather than to wish for medicines'
Thomas More, Utopia, 1516

Primary prevention

Cancer is not caused by one factor but is multi-factorial. Causes include the following:

- Lifestyle exposures, e.g. obesity, alcohol, smoking, and viruses
- Environmental exposures, e.g. Asbestos, azo dyes, radiation exposure
- Inherited genetic susceptibility, e.g. *BRCA 1* and *2* (account for 2%–5% of all breast cancers).

Current thinking suggests that 90% of all cancers may have a lifestyle or environmental trigger, and thus may be preventable. The trigger causes deoxyribonucleic acid (DNA) damage, and may occur many years before the appearance of the tumour. The tumour only appears when the 'initiated' cells proliferate by a process known as 'promotion'.

Primary and secondary prevention: *Primary prevention* aims to modify factors that promote or protect against carcinogenesis. *Secondary prevention* aims to detect pre-malignant disease or early malignant disease at a stage when it is still curable.

Primary prevention strategies

Dietary modification: There is a substantial body of evidence that links diet to cancer risk. For example, colorectal cancer is more common in a population having a low-fibre diet, high in animal fats and protein, and low in fresh fruit and vegetables. Some food additives are known carcinogens and have been banned from use. There is some evidence that diets rich in anti-oxidants may reduce cancer risk. Furthermore, obesity is associated with increased risk of breast, endometrial, colorectal, and renal cancers.

Smoking cessation: Smoking (both direct and passive exposure) is associated with increased rates of lung cancer, lip and other mouth and throat cancers, stomach cancer, colorectal cancer, and bladder cancer. Smoking cessation reduces risk of cancer.

Alcohol reduction: Excess alcohol intake is particularly associated with liver cancer and oropharyngeal cancers. It is also associated with breast cancer and oesophageal cancer.

Awareness and avoidance of occupational carcinogens: Mesothelioma can follow even minimal exposure to asbestos. There may be a long time lag of 20–40y between exposure and disease but mean time to death following diagnosis is just 2y. Workers exposed to asbestos also have increased risk of adenocarcinoma of the lung, stomach, and colo-rectum. Smokers exposed to asbestos have 5× ↑ risk of lung cancer compared to non-smokers exposed to asbestos.

Other cancers associated with occupation include the following:

- Woodworkers—nasal cancer
- Polyvinyl chloride (PVC) manufacturers—liver cancer
- Nickel refiners—lung and nasal cancer
- Azo-dye manufacturers—bladder cancer

Reducing sun exposure: Sun exposure is a major risk factor for basal and squamous cell skin cancer and malignant melanoma. Risk of skin cancer can be reduced by adhering to the Sun Safety Code.

Vaccinating against virus-related cancers: Several viral infections are known to cause cancer. These include:

- Hepatitis B and C—associated with liver cancer
- HIV—associated classically with Kaposi's sarcoma and lymphoma, but ↑ the risk of many tumours
- Epstein–Barr virus—associated with Burkitt lymphoma, nasopharyngeal carcinoma, and lymphoma
- HPV—associated with cervical, vulvo-vaginal, anal, and some oropharyngeal cancers.

Where vaccines are available, vaccination against carcinogenic viral infection may prevent cancer. In the UK high-risk infants are vaccinated against Hepatitis B. HPV vaccines are aimed at preventing infection with strains causing cervical cancer. Currently vaccines are available that target strains 16 and 18 which account for ~70% of HPV-related cancer cases ± strains 6 and 11. Vaccination will be targeted at girls before the age at which they become sexually active (~11y). Cervical screening is still necessary as the vaccine does not protect against all strains causing cervical cancer.

Avoiding high-risk sexual activity: Avoidance of high-risk sexual activity reduces the risk of HPV, Hepatitis B and HIV infection (see above).

Surgical prevention: Certain cancers associated with congenital/genetic abnormalities (e.g. undescended testes, ulcerative colitis, familial adenomatous polyposis (FAP), other hereditary colorectal cancers, ovarian cancer, breast cancer) may be prevented by prophylactic surgery.

Genetic screening: In 2003, the Human Genome Project revealed the DNA sequence for 30,000 genes. Despite these advances, the impact of lifestyle and environmental factors which lead to genetic mutations make determining an individual's risk of cancer from a 'genetic blueprint' extremely difficult. However, genes predicting some forms of cancer have been identified—particularly genes predicting breast and ovarian cancer. Trials of primary prevention for women at high genetic risk of breast cancer are underway. Consider referral if high genetic risk of breast cancer (Figure 2.4, 🕮 p.27)

Advice for patients

Prevention of skin cancer: The Sun Safety Code:

- Take care not to burn in the sun
- Cover up with loose cool clothing, a hat, and sun glasses
- If you're swimming outdoors or on the beach, wear an ultraviolet (UV) protective sunsuit (especially important for children). When out of the water, add a T-shirt, sunglasses, and sunhat
- Seek shade during the hottest part of the day
- Apply a high-factor sunscreen on any parts of the body exposed to the sun (≥sun protection factor [SPF] 25).

Information for patients on preventing sunburn:

Cancer Research UK Sun Smart Campaign
🖥 www.cancerresearchuk.org/SunSmart

Secondary prevention

The idea of cancer screening is attractive—the ability to diagnose and treat a potentially serious condition at an early stage when it is still treatable. An ideal screening test should pick up all those who have the disease (have high sensitivity) and must exclude those who do not (high specificity). It must detect *only* those who have a disease (high positive predictive value) and should exclude *only* those who do not have the disease (high negative predictive value)—Table 2.1.

Wilson–Jungner criteria*: All screening tests should meet the following criteria before they are introduced to the target population:
- The condition must be an important health problem
- Natural history of the condition must be well understood
- There must be a detectable early stage
- Treatment at early stage must be of more benefit than at late stage
- There must be a suitable test to detect early stage disease
- The test must be acceptable to the target population
- Intervals for repeating the test must have been determined
- Adequate health service provision must have been made for the extra-clinical workload resulting from screening
- Risks, both physical and psychological, must be less than benefits
- Costs must be worthwhile in relation to benefits gained.

Screening programme effectiveness: For a screening programme to be effective and ↓ morbidity and mortality there must be:
- Adequate participation of the target population
- Few false negative or false positive results (Table 2.1)
- Screening intervals shorter than the time taken for the disease to develop to an untreatable stage.
- Adequate follow-up of all abnormal results.
- Effective treatment at the stage detected by screening.

Further information:
National Electronic Library for Screening ▣ www.library.nhs.uk/screening
NHS Cancer Screening Programmes ▣ www.cancerscreening.nhs.uk

GP notes

Cancer screening: There is no ideal screening test. Always explain:
- Purpose of screening
- Likelihood of positive/negative findings and possibility of false positive/negative results
- Uncertainties and risks attached to the screening process (Table 2.2)
- Significant medical, social or financial implications of screening for the particular condition or predisposition
- Follow-up plans, including availability of counselling and support services.

Table 2.1 Performance of screening tests

		Disease	
		Present	Absent
Test	Positive	True positive (a)	False positive (b)
	Negative	False negative (c)	True negative (d)

Sensitivity = $a/(a + c)$; Negative predictive value = $d/(c + d)$
Specificity = $d/(b + d)$; Positive predictive value = $a/(a + b)$

Table 2.2 Pros and cons of cancer screening

Benefits	Disadvantages
• Improved prognosis for some cases detected by screening	• Longer morbidity in cases where prognosis is unaltered
• Less radical treatment for some early cases	• Overtreatment of questionable abnormalities
• Reassurance for those with negative test results	• False reassurance for those with false negative results
• Increased information on natural history of disease and benefits of treatment at early stage.	• Anxiety and sometimes morbidity for those with false positive results
	• Unnecessary intervention for those with false positive results
	• Hazard of screening test
	• Diversion of resources to the screening programme.

Cervical cancer screening

Screening prevents ~1,000–4,000 deaths/y in the UK from squamous cell cancer of the cervix (Figure 2.1). Cervical cancer almost exclusively occurs in women who are or have been sexually active.

Liquidbased cytology: In the UK, the traditional Papanicolou smear (Pap smear) has been replaced by liquid based cytology. The sample is collected in a similar way but, rather than smearing the sample from the spatula onto a slide, the head of the spatula, where the cells are lodged, is broken off or raised into a vial containing preservative fluid. This method ↓ the number of inadequate smears taken as cervical cells can be examined even if the sample is contaminated with blood, pus, or mucus.

Taking a smear: Ensure adequate training—poor smear taking misses 20% abnormalities. Courses are available—update skills every 3y. Give all women information about the test, condition being sought, possible results of screening, and their implications.

Timing: Avoid menstruation if possible (note on the request form if unavoidable). Ideal time is mid-cycle. Routine bimanual examination is unnecessary—do a pelvic examination only if clinically indicated (e.g. painful/heavy periods).

Screening interval: A smear test is routinely offered to all women aged 25–64y who are sexually active. There is no upper age limit for the first smear. Frequency of screening depends on age:

- 25–49y   Three yearly screening intervals.
- 50–64y   Five yearly screening intervals.
- 65y +   Only screen those who have not been screened since age 50y or have had recent abnormal tests.

Organization of the cervical screening programme: Practices undertaking cervical screening must:
- Provide information to eligible women to allow them to make an informed decision about taking part in the programme
- Perform the cervical screening test (and ensure staff are properly trained and equipped to perform the test)
- Arrange for women to be informed about the results of their tests (unless this is automatically done by the laboratory)
- Ensure that results are followed up appropriately *and*
- Maintain records of tests carried out, results, and any clinical follow-up requirements (Table 2.3).

The role of HPV testing: Infection with HPV 16, 18, 31, and 33 is associated with CIN/cervical cancer. 99.7% of cervical cancers contain HPV DNA and women with HPV infection are 70× more likely to develop high-grade cervical abnormalities. A pilot of HPV testing is being conducted within the UK cervical screening programme. Women with borderline/mild dyskaryosis are tested for high-risk HPV (using the sample collected for cytology). If HPV is found, the patient is referred to colposcopy; if HPV is not found the patient is invited for a repeat smear and further HPV test after 6mo.

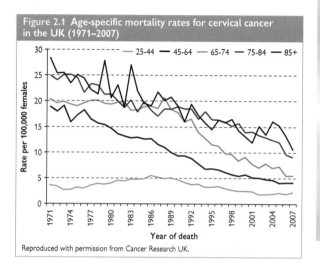

Figure 2.1 Age-specific mortality rates for cervical cancer in the UK (1971–2007)

Reproduced with permission from Cancer Research UK.

GMS contract			
Cervical screening 1	% of patients aged 25–64y (21–60y in Scotland) whose notes confirm that a cervical smear has been performed in the last 5y.	Up to 11 points	40%–80%
Cervical screening 5	The practice has a system of informing all women of the results of cervical smears.	2 points	
Cervical screening 6	The practice has a policy for auditing its cervical screening service and performs an audit of inadequate smears in relation to individual smear takers at least every 2y.	2 points	
Cervical screening 7	The practice has a protocol that is in line with national guidance and practice for the management of cervical screening, which includes staff training, management of patient call/recall, exception reporting, and the regular monitoring of inadequate smear rates.	7 points	

GMS practices are expected to perform cervical screening for all women aged 25–64y (21–60y in Scotland) registered with the practice as an additional service. Opting out results in a 1.1% ↓ in the global sum payment.

Table 2.3 Interpretation of smear results and action

Result	What does it mean?	Action
Normal	No nuclear abnormalities.	Place on routine recall.
Inadequate (~9% conventional smears; ~2% with liquid based cytology)	Insufficient material present or poorly spread/fixed. Vision of cells obscured by debris.	Repeat the smear as soon as convenient. After three consecutive inadequate results, refer for colposcopy.
Borderline dyskaryosis (5%–10% smears are borderline or mild)	Some nuclear abnormalities but not clear whether these changes represent dyskaryosis.	Repeat smear every 6mo. Most changes will have reverted to normal. After three consecutive normal smears, return to normal recall. If abnormality persists 3×, or worsens, refer for colposcopy. If in a 10y period there are three borderline or more severe results, refer for colposcopy.
Mild dyskaryosis (5%–10% smears are borderline or mild)	Nuclear abnormalities indicative of low-grade CIN.	Repeat smear every 6mo. Most changes will have reverted to normal. After three consecutive normal smears, return to normal recall. If abnormality persists ×2, refer for colposcopy. If in a 10y period there are three mild or more severe results, refer for colposcopy. If CIN1 is confirmed on colposcopy, management options are to watch and wait (three normal smears 6mo apart are needed before return to normal recall) or treat.*
Moderate dyskaryosis (1% smears)	Nuclear abnormalities reflecting probable CIN2.	Refer to colposcopy. If CIN is confirmed on colposcopy, treat.*
Severe dyskaryosis or worse (0.6% smears)	Nuclear abnormalities reflecting probable CIN3.	Refer to colposcopy or (rarely) make referral to gynaecological oncologist if invasive carcinoma is suspected. If CIN is confirmed on colposcopy, treat.*

Other possible abnormalities seen on cervical smear
- Dyskaryotic glandular cells—refer for colposcopy.
- Atrophic—common in peri-/post-menopausal women. No action.
- Endometrial cells—may be normal if IUCD in situ, hormonal treatment or first half of 28d-cycle. Otherwise, discuss with laboratory. Refer if reported as abnormal.
- Inflammatory changes—common finding. Take chlamydial, endocervical, and high-vaginal swabs. Treat as necessary.
- Trichomonas, Candida, or changes associated with herpes simplex virus (HSV) infection—Treat trichomonas or candida. Discuss any new diagnosis of HSV with the patient.
- Actinomyces—Associated with IUCDs.

* Following treatment women with high-grade disease (CIN2, CIN3, and cervical glandular intra-epithelial neoplasia [cGIN]) require a smear at 6mo and 12mo then annually for at least 9y. Women treated for low-grade disease require a smear at 6mo, 12mo, and 24mo.

Advice for patients: Advice and support

Frequently asked questions about cervical screening:

Should I have cervical screening if I'm pregnant or trying to get pregnant? Ideally women should not have cervical screening when pregnant or possibly pregnant. However, this will depend on your own individual circumstances. If you've had abnormal smears in the past, for example, or if you haven't accepted your past invitations for screening, then you should consult your doctor or practice nurse to ask for advice. If you have a normal smear history then it's better to wait until about 3 months after the delivery before you go for cervical screening.

When is the best time in the menstrual cycle to have cervical screening? Mid-cycle (usually between 10 and 16 days after your last period) is the best time because a clearer sample can be obtained around this time. But it's not a strict rule, so do take advice from your doctor or practice nurse if you can't make an appointment at that time.

Will cervical screening pick up any other infections? It might, but that's not really the aim of the programme which is to detect and treat early abnormalities which, if left untreated, could lead to cervical cancer. Incidental findings of infections may be reported. Your doctor will then act on them as needed.

I've had a hysterectomy—do I still need cervical screening? If your cervix is still present after your hysterectomy then you will still need cervical smears. Sometimes another sort of smear (a vault smear) is needed after hysterectomy even if you don't have a cervix. Normally, if you do not have a cervix, then you do not need cervical screening. The surgical team who performed the operation will decide what kind of follow-up is appropriate.

My cervical screening test showed borderline changes. Why do I have to wait 6 months for a repeat test—won't they get worse? The reason we repeat the test in 6 months is to give minor changes a chance to get better without any treatment which is usually what happens. If the repeat test is normal, you will be asked to have two more tests in 6 and 12 months time to check that the cells are still healthy. You can then go back to receiving routine invitations as before. If your repeat test still shows borderline changes (also called mild dyskaryosis), you may be referred for a colposcopy.

Further information for patients:

Cervical Screening—the Facts 🖳 www.cancerscreening.org.uk

Reproduced with permission in modified format from 🖳 www.cancerscreening.nhs.uk.

Further information:
NHS Cervical Screening: 🖳 www.cancerscreening.org.uk
Cancer Research UK Cervical Screening 🖳
www.cancerresearch.org.uk/cancerstats

Breast cancer screening

In the UK there has been a national screening programme for breast cancer since 1988. The aim of the programme is to detect breast cancer at an early stage in order to ↑ survival chances (Stage I tumours—5y survival, 84%; Stage IV tumours—5y survival, 18%)—Figure 2.2.

Breast awareness: Trials of self-examination have not demonstrated ↓ mortality. Instead less formal 'Breast Awareness' is advocated.

Screening test

Women >50y 2-view mammographic screening is currently available to women aged 50–70y every 3 y. This is soon to be extended to women aged 47–73y. Older women can also request screening every 3y. Screening detects 85% of cancers in women aged >50y (60% of which are impalpable) and ~ 70–80% screening-detected cancers have good prognosis. Screening more frequently does not ↓ mortality[R]. Organization of breast cancer screening in the UK—Figure 2.3.

High risk women <50y Women with family history of breast cancer may be at ↑ risk of breast cancer themselves (Figure 2.4, 📖 p.27) and may benefit from earlier screening and/or genetic screening:

- All raised/high risk women aged 40–49y—should be offered annual 2-view mammography
- Women known to have a genetic mutation should be offered annual MRI surveillance - from 20y if TP53 mutation, and from 30y if BRCA1/2 mutation.
- MRI surveillance should also be offered to women aged 30–39y with 10y risk >8%; women aged 40–49y with 10y risk >20%; and at risk women aged 40–49y with a dense breast pattern on mammography

Interval cancers Cancer developing in the interval between screens. In the first year after screening, 20% breast cancers are interval cancers. This ↑ to ~ 60% in the 3rd year.

Acceptability of screening 81% women find mammography uncomfortable but 90% return for subsequent screens. GPs have an important role—sending personalized invitations for screening to women from their GPs increases uptake rates[®].

Anxiety due to screening False positive results cause anxiety as well as prompting further invasive investigations. Anxiety levels in women recalled and then found to be disease-free are higher in year after the recall appointment, than in women who receive negative results at screening.

Further information
NHS Breast Screening 🖳 www.cancerscreening.nhs.uk
NICE Familial breast cancer (2006) 🖳 www.nice.org.uk

Information for patients 🖳 www.cancerscreening.nhs.uk
- Breast Screening—the Facts
- Over 70? You are still entitled to breast screening

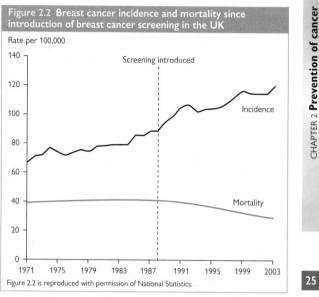

Figure 2.2 Breast cancer incidence and mortality since introduction of breast cancer screening in the UK

Rate per 100,000

Screening introduced

Incidence

Mortality

Figure 2.2 is reproduced with permission of National Statistics.

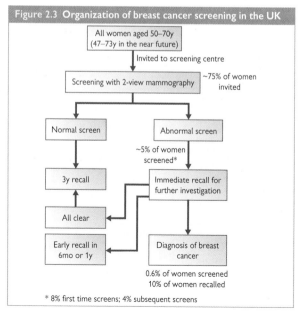

Figure 2.3 Organization of breast cancer screening in the UK

All women aged 50–70y (47–73y in the near future)

Invited to screening centre

Screening with 2-view mammography

~75% of women invited

Normal screen

Abnormal screen

~5% of women screened*

3y recall

Immediate recall for further investigation

All clear

Early recall in 6mo or 1y

Diagnosis of breast cancer

0.6% of women screened
10% of women recalled

* 8% first time screens; 4% subsequent screens

Advice for patients

Frequently asked questions about breast cancer screening:

I haven't been called for breast screening even though I'm over 50—do I need to contact anyone? The National Health Service (NHS) Breast Screening Programme is a rolling one which calls women from doctors' practices in turn. This means not every woman receives her invitation as soon as she is 50. It will be sometime between the ages of 49 and 52. If you are registered with a GP and the practice has your correct details, then you will automatically receive an invitation. You don't need to contact anyone but you might like to check your surgery has your correct contact details and ask them when the women on their list are next due for screening.

I'm worried that I might have breast cancer. Can I walk into the mobile breast screening unit and request a mammogram? The NHS Breast Screening Programme is a population screening programme that invites all women aged 50–70 as a matter of routine. It is not aimed at women who already have symptoms. So if you have found something that worries you or are concerned about your breast health, you should see your GP in the usual way. He or she will decide whether or not you need to be referred for further investigations or treatment.

Why doesn't the NHS screen younger women? Mammograms are not as effective in younger women because the density of the breast tissue makes it more difficult to detect problems and also because the incidence of breast cancer is lower at this age. The average age of the menopause in the UK is 50 and so this is the age when women join the NHS Breast Screening Programme. As women go past the menopause, the glandular tissue in their breast reduces and the breast tissue is increasingly made up of only fat. This is clearer on the mammogram and makes interpretation more reliable.

Why does breast screening stop at 70? It doesn't. Although women over 70 are not routinely invited for breast screening, they are encouraged to call the local unit to request breast screening every 3 years. Cards have been produced to help them remember and these are handed out at their last routine breast screening appointment.

Women abroad get more frequent breast screening. Why doesn't this happen in the UK? A large research trial in 2002 concluded that the NHS Breast Screening Programme has got the interval between screening and invitations about right at 3 years, compared with more frequent screening.

Frequently asked questions are reproduced with permission in modified format from 🖫 http://www.cancerscreening.org.uk/breastscreen/faqs.html

Further information:

Breast Screening—the Facts—available from 🖫 www.cancerscreening.org.uk
Over 70? You are still entitled to breast screening—available from 🖫 www.cancerscreening.org.uk

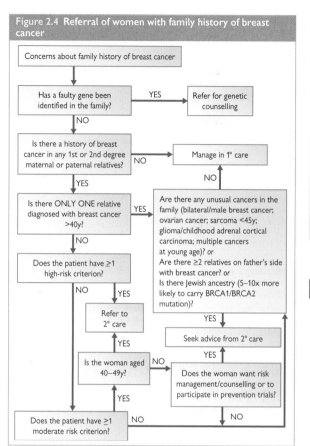

Figure 2.4 Referral of women with family history of breast cancer

Concerns about family history of breast cancer

Has a faulty gene been identified in the family? → YES → Refer for genetic counselling

NO

Is there a history of breast cancer in any 1st or 2nd degree maternal or paternal relatives? → NO → Manage in 1° care

YES

Is there ONLY ONE relative diagnosed with breast cancer >40y? → YES → Are there any unusual cancers in the family (bilateral/male breast cancer; ovarian cancer; sarcoma <45y; glioma/childhood adrenal cortical carcinoma; multiple cancers at young age)? or Are there ≥2 relatives on father's side with breast cancer? or Is there Jewish ancestry (5–10x more likely to carry BRCA1/BRCA2 mutation)?

NO

Does the patient have ≥1 high-risk criterion?

NO / YES

Refer to 2° care

Seek advice from 2° care

Is the woman aged 40–49y? → NO → Does the woman want risk management/counselling or to participate in prevention trials?

YES

Does the patient have ≥1 moderate risk criterion? → NO

High-risk criteria

Female breast cancer:
1× 1st degree relative + 1× 2nd degree relative diagnosed < average age of 50y.
2× 1st degree relatives diagnosed < average age of 50y.
1× 1st degree relative with bilateral breast cancer where first primary diagnosed at <50y.
≥3× 1st/2nd degree relatives.
Male breast cancer: 1× 1st degree relative.
Breast and ovarian cancer: 1× 1st/2nd degree relative with breast cancer + another with ovarian cancer (1 must be 1st degree relative).

Moderate-risk criteria

Female breast cancer:
1× 1st degree relative <40y.
1× 1st degree relative + 1× 2nd degree relative diagnosed > average age of 50y.
2× 1st degree relatives diagnosed > average age of 50y.

1st degree relative—mother, father, sister, brother, daughter, son.

2nd degree relative—grandparents, grandchildren, aunt, uncle, niece, nephew, half-sister/brother.

Colorectal cancer screening

Screening for colorectal cancer started in the UK in 2009. Patients presenting with tumour confined to the bowel wall have >90% long-term survival. However, without screening, most tumours are detected at advanced stages and overall 5y survival is ≈40%. The aim of the programme is to detect colorectal cancer at an early stage to ↑ survival chances.

Screening test: Information for patients—📖 p.30
- Faecal occult blood (FOB) testing kits are sent every 2y to all patients aged 60–69y with instructions for completion at home and return. Patients >70y may also request testing kits
- The test kit has three flaps, each with two windows underneath. Two samples are taken from a bowel motion and spread onto the two windows under the first flap using the cardboard sticks provided. The flap is then sealed and the process repeated using the remaining two flaps for the subsequent two bowel motions
- Once all six windows have been used, the kit is returned. Kits must be returned <14d after the first sample is taken
- A result is then sent to the patient in <2wk

Screening outcomes: Tables 2.4 and 2.5. It is estimated that ~2% of those tested will be referred on for colonoscopy, and if 60% of those aged 60–69y do the FOB test, 1,200 deaths will be prevented each year.

Family history: If a patient has one first-degree relative (mother, father, sister, brother, daughter, or son) with colorectal cancer, risk of developing colorectal cancer is ↑ ×2–3.

Refer for colonoscopy at presentation or aged 35–40y (whichever is later) and repeat colonoscopy aged 55y if:
- 2× first-degree relatives with a history of colorectal cancer *or*
- 1× first-degree relative with a history of colorectal cancer aged <45y.

Refer for specialist follow-up and genetic counselling if:
- >2× first-degree relatives with a history of colorectal cancer or
- Family history of:
  - Familial adenomatous polyposis (FAP)
  - Juvenile polyposis
  - Peutz–Jehger syndrome
  - Hereditary non-polyposis colorectal cancer
  - MMR oncogene

Ulcerative colitis: Patients with ulcerative colitis have ↑ risk of colorectal cancer. Offer all patients a follow-up plan agreed with their specialist. In some cases, prophylactic colectomy is appropriate.

Previous colorectal cancer: Patients with history of previous colorectal cancer are at ↑ risk of developing a second colorectal primary. After successful treatment, younger patients are routinely followed up with colonoscopy every 5y until 70y In primary care, even if secondary care monitoring is in progress, remain vigilant for recurrences and re-refer urgently if suspected.

Table 2.4 Screening outcomes

FOB result	Explanation	Action
Normal	0 +ve spots	Screening offered again in 2y if <70y.
Unclear ~4% tested	1–4 +ve spots	Test repeated if If the second test is abnormal colonoscopy is offered If the second test is normal, a third test is requested. If the third test is normal repeat screening in 2y is offered if <70y If the third test is abnormal, colonoscopy is offered.
Abnormal	5–6 +ve spots	Colonoscopy is offered.
Technical failure	Laboratory error	Repeat testing is offered.
Spoilt kit	Patient error	Repeat testing is offered.

Table 2.5 Colonoscopy outcomes

- Uptake of colonoscopy following abnormal FOB testing is ~80%.
- Sensitivity of colonoscopy to detect significant abnormalities is ~90%.
- Polyps found during colonoscopy are usually removed.
- Complications of colonoscopy include heavy bleeding (1:150); bowel perforation (1:1,500); death (1:10,000).

Normal (50%)		No abnormalities detected.	FOB screening offered again in 2y if <70y.
Polyp (40%)	Low risk	1–2 small (<1cm) adenomas	FOB screening offered again in 2y if <70y.
	Intermediate risk	3–4 small (<1cm) adenomas or ≥1 adenoma ≥1cm	Three yearly colonoscopy until 2× negative examinations.
	High risk	≥five adenomas or ≥three adenomas of which at least 1 is ≥1cm	Colonoscopy at 12mo then three yearly colonoscopy until 2× negative examinations.
Cancer (10%)		Colorectal cancer detected at colonoscopy.	Refer urgently for further treatment.
Other pathology		Other pathology (e.g. UC) detected at colonoscopy.	Refer/treat/advise as necessary.
Technical difficulty (5%)		Unable to negotiate the colonoscope around the bowel.	Repeat colonoscopy or alternative imaging.

Further information:

NICE Referral guidelines for suspected cancer—quick reference guide (2005) www.nice.org.uk
NHS Bowel Cancer Screening Programme www.cancerscreening.nhs.uk

Advice for patients

Frequently asked questions about bowel cancer screening:

What is the purpose of bowel cancer screening? Bowel cancer screening aims to detect cancer of the colon or rectum at an early stage, before there are any symptoms, when treatment is more likely to be effective.

Is screening for bowel cancer important? Approximately 1 in 20 people in the UK will develop colorectal cancer during their lifetime. It is the third most common cancer in the UK, and causes 16,000 deaths each year in the UK. Regular screening has been shown to reduce the risk of dying from colorectal cancer by 16%.

What does the NHS Bowel Cancer Screening Programme do? This programme offers screening every 2 years to all men and women between the ages of 60–69 in the UK. Invitations are automatically sent to everyone in this age group along with a screening kit so that they can do the test at home. The test involves taking a small amount of your bowel motion and putting it on a card. Although some might find this test unpleasant, it can be done in the privacy of your own home.

If you are aged 70 or over, you can ask for a screening kit by calling freephone number: 0800 707 60 60

What happens if I have an abnormal result? Depending on the result of your test, you may be asked to repeat the test, and/or be referred for a colonoscopy. A colonoscopy is an investigation which involves looking at your bowel directly with a telescope. Most people who are offered colonoscopy will not have cancer, but in the unlikely event that colonoscopy shows that you do have bowel cancer, you will be referred immediately for specialist treatment. If bowel cancer is picked up at the earliest stage, you have a 90% chance of survival.

Does screening pick up all colorectal cancers? No test is 100% accurate. There is a small possibility that you can have a negative screening test and still have bowel cancer. Stay alert to symptoms of bowel cancer and see your GP if you are worried. Symptoms to look out for are:
- Change in bowel habit—particularly diarrhoea for several weeks
- Bleeding from your back passage without any obvious reason
- Abdominal pain—particularly if it is severe
- A lump in your abdomen.

Further information for patients:

Bowel cancer screening—the Facts 🖳 www.cancerscreening.nhs.uk

Reproduced in modified format with permission from the NHS Bowel Cancer Screening Programme

Advice for patients: Taking the prostate-specific antigen test

What is prostate cancer? The prostate gland lies beneath the bladder. Each year in the UK approximately 22,000 men are diagnosed with prostate cancer and 9500 die from the disease. Prostate cancer is rare in men below the age of 50 years, and the average age of diagnosis is 75 years. Slow-growing cancers are more common than fast-growing cancers and may not cause any symptoms or shorten life.

What is the PSA test? Prostate-specific antigen (PSA) is a substance produced by the prostate gland. The PSA test is a blood test. If the levels of PSA in the blood are raised, it can give an early indication that prostate cancer is present. This test is now available to men who wish to be tested.

What if the test comes back normal? You are unlikely to have cancer. However, the PSA test can miss prostate cancer. If you have urinary symptoms, consult your GP.

What if the PSA levels are raised? The higher the level of PSA in the blood, the more likely it is to be cancer, but there are other causes of raised PSA levels too—for instance, enlargement of the prostate, and prostate or urine infection. Roughly two-thirds of men with raised PSA levels will *not* have prostate cancer. Your GP will examine you to check your prostate gland and will either refer you to a specialist or repeat the PSA test in a few months.

What happens when you have been referred to a specialist? The specialist usually performs a prostate biopsy to determine if prostate cancer is present. This involves taking samples from the prostate through the back passage. Most men find this uncomfortable. Sometimes complications or infection may occur. Roughly 2 out of 3 men who have a prostate biopsy will not have prostate cancer. However, biopsies can miss some cancers and worry about prostate cancer may remain even after a clear result. Treatment depends on your age and the biopsy results.

So, should I have the PSA test? That is your decision.

Benefits of PSA testing	Downside of PSA testing
• It may provide reassurance if the test result is normal	• It can miss cancer, and provide false reassurance
• It may find cancer before symptoms develop	• It may lead to unnecessary anxiety and medical tests when no cancer is present
• It may detect cancer at an early stage when treatments could be beneficial	• It might detect slow-growing cancer that may never cause any symptoms or shortened life span
• If treatment is successful, the consequences of more advanced cancer are avoided.	• The main treatments of prostate cancer have significant side effects, and there is no certainty that the treatment will be successful.

Patient information is reproduced from *PSA testing for prostate cancer* with permission from the NHS Cancer Screening Programme.

31

Prostate cancer screening

Prostate cancer is the second most common cancer worldwide. In the UK, it is the most common cancer affecting men and 10,000 men die from the disease every year. 1:10 men have clinical prostate cancer in their lifetimes and the incidence is rising. A large-scale trial of screening for prostate cancer is underway in the UK.

Problems with screening:

- Incidental post-mortem evidence of prostate cancer is high (≈75% men >75y) and very few become clinically evident, so many more men would be found with prostate cancer by screening than would die or have symptoms from it
- Natural history of prostate cancer is not understood—there is no means to detect which 'early' cancers become more widespread
- Inadequate screening tests (see below)
- It is not clear if early treatment enhances life expectancy
- Peak incidence of morbidity and mortality is in old age (75–79y) so potential years of life saved by screening are small.

Screening tests:

- PSA: See below.
- Digital rectal examination (DRE): Operator-dependant, fails to detect early prostate cancers, and lacks specificity. Annual screening in the US and Germany has not ↓ mortality.
- Transrectal ultrasound (TRUS): Too expensive for widespread use.

The most effective screening regime involves rectal examination and PSA testing followed by TRUS for suspicious lesions[S]. Optimal screening interval is unknown but serial screening does ↑ detection.

PSA testing: There is considerable demand for PSA testing amongst men worried about prostate cancer. The Government has introduced a PSA Informed Choice Programme under which men can request a PSA test. Patients should be warned about the poor specificity of the test before performing the test and information about the pros and cons of testing should also be provided. In addition, PSA is routinely measured in men with urological symptoms. Abnormal PSA is a common reason for referral to an urologist. Its sensitivity and specificity are poor (Table 2.6).

Performing a PSA test: Do the PSA test before doing a DRE. If that is not possible, delay the test for 1wk after the examination. Exclude urinary infection before PSA testing. Do NOT do a PSA test if the man has:
- A proven UTI—treat the UTI and postpone the PSA test for ≥1mo
- Ejaculated within 48h
- Exercised vigorously in the previous 48h
- Had a prostate biopsy <6wk ago.

Reasons for increased PSA:
- Prostate cancer
- Benign prostatic hypertrophy
- Acute or chronic prostatitis
- Physical exercise
- Acute urinary retention

- Prostate instrumentation (includes prostate biopsy, urinary catheterization and rectal examination)
- Old age

❶ PSA may be *normal* when early prostate cancer is present.

Further information:
NICE 🖥 www.nice.org.uk
- Improving outcomes in urological cancers (2002)
- Referral guidelines for suspected cancer (2005)

Cancer research UK 🖥 www.cancerresearchuk.org
National screening 🖥 www.cancerscreening.nhs.uk

Table 2.6 **PSA cut offs which should prompt referral**	
Age (y)	Refer to urology if PSA (ng/ml)
50–59	≥3.0
60–69	≥4.0
≥70	>5.0
❶ Finasteride ↓ PSA by ~5%	

Advice for patients

Further information about PSA testing and prostate cancer:

National screening 🖥 www.cancerscreening.nhs.uk
Patient experience database 🖥 www.healthtalkonline.org
Macmillan Cancer Support ☎ 0808 808 0000 🖥 www.macmillan.org.uk
Prostate cancer charity ☎ 0800 074 8383 🖥 www.prostate-cancer.org.uk
Prostate cancer support association ☎ 0845 601 0766 🖥 www.prostatecancersupport.co.uk

Chapter 3

Diagnosis of cancer

35

Assessment of suspected cancer

Early detection of cancer is crucial to improve patients' chances of survival. Unfortunately early signs of cancer are often easier to see with the benefit of hindsight, than they are at the time of presentation.

The challenge of detecting cancer: Although cancer is common, cancer diagnosis is a relatively rare occurrence for an individual GP. Referral from primary to secondary care is often triggered by a GP's awareness of 'alarm symptoms' or 'red flags' that are considered to predict malignant disease.

General assessment: Objectives are to:
- Establish a constructive relationship with the patient to enable patient and doctor to communicate effectively and serve as the basis for any subsequent therapeutic relationship
- Find out whether the patient has any predisposing factors to a diagnosis of cancer
- Determine whether the patient has alarm symptoms that might suggest a diagnosis of cancer and, if so, what they are
- Assess the patient's emotions and attitudes towards the problem
- Establish the best course of action.

History: Use open questions at the start becoming directive when necessary—clarify, reflect, facilitate, listen. *Ask about:*

Presenting complaint: Chronological account, specific symptoms, past history of similar symptoms. Be alert to a possible diagnosis of cancer when a patient presents with non-specific symptoms/signs such as:
- Anorexia and/or weight loss for no apparent reason
- Malaise/lethargy with no apparent cause
- Fever/sweats
- Generalized itching
- Breathlessness
- Bone pain
- Lymphadenopathy
- Recurrent infections/failure to recover as expected.

Specific alarm symptoms/signs: 🕮 p.38–48

Past medical history: Previous malignancy, previous radiotherapy, or chemotherapy, conditions predisposing to cancer e.g. ulcerative colitis (UC), abnormal smears.

Social history: Could occupation predispose to malignancy (e.g. asbestos worker)? Smoker? Housing, social support etc.

Family history: Any family history of cancer.

Attitudes and beliefs: How does the patient see the problem? What does he think is wrong?

Examination: Tailor to symptoms reported and suspected diagnosis.

Action:
- Summarize the history back to the patient and give an opportunity for the patient to fill in any gaps
- Outline a management plan
- Set a review date.

Speed of referral: All 'urgent' referrals for suspected cancer should be made <1 working day after the decision to refer, and seen by a specialist in <2wk from the date of referral.

Significant event audit (critical event monitoring): This is a recognized methodology for reflecting on important events in a practice. New diagnoses of cancer are suitable topics for significant event audits. For it to be effective, it must be practised in a culture that avoids blame and involves all disciplines. There are three steps:

- *Decide on a topic and plan a meeting*
- At the end of the discussion *come to a decision* about the case e.g. well managed, need change in procedure etc.
- *Prepare a report.* The two acceptable formats for laying out these reports are described in Table 3.1.

Further information:

BMJ Jones *et al.* Alarm symptoms in early diagnosis of cancer in primary care: cohort study using General Practice Research Database (2007) **334**: 1040

NICE Referral guidelines for suspected cancer—quick reference guide (2005) 🖳 www.nice.org.uk

Table 3.1 Methods of reporting significant event audits

Reporting method 1	Reporting method 2
Description of event—brief. Can be in note form.	*What happened?*
Learning outcome—aspects of high standard and those which could be improved. Where appropriate include why the event occurred.	*Why did it happen?*
	Was insight demonstrated?
Action plan—decision(s) taken. Describe reasons for decisions together with any other lessons learned from the discussion.	*Was change implemented?*

GMS contract

Cancer 1	The practice can produce a register of all cancer patients, excluding non-melanotic skin cancer, from 1.4.2003.	5	
Cancer 3	% of patients with cancer, diagnosed <18mo ago who have a patient review recorded as occurring <6mo after the practice received confirmation of diagnosis.	6	40%–90%
Education 7	The practice has undertaken ≥12 significant event reviews in the past 3y which could include new cancer diagnoses.	4 points for 12 reviews	
Education 10	The practice has undertaken ≥3 significant event reviews within the last year.	6 points for 3 reviews	

Suspected brain, head, or neck cancer

Headache: If new, unexplained headaches, undertake a neurological examination guided by the symptoms, but including examination for papilloedema.

ⓘ Absence of papilloedema does not exclude brain tumour.

Refer urgently to neurology/neurosurgery/brain imaging if:
- Headache in a patient in whom a brain tumour is suspected
- Headaches of recent onset accompanied by features suggestive of raised intra-cranial pressure, for example:
  - Vomiting
  - Drowsiness
  - Posture-related headache
  - Pulse-synchronous tinnitus

or by other focal or non-focal neurological symptoms, for example, blackout, change in personality or memory
- A new, qualitatively different, unexplained headache that becomes progressively severe
- Persistent headache if past history of any cancer.

Consider non-urgent referral or discussion with specialist: For all patients with unexplained headaches of recent onset:
- Present for at ≥1mo *and*
- Not accompanied by features suggestive of ↑ intra-cranial pressure.

Other neurological symptoms: Undertake a neurological examination guided by the symptoms, but including examination for papilloedema. ⓘ Absence of papilloedema does not exclude brain tumour.

Refer urgently to neurology/neurosurgery/brain imaging if:
- Symptoms related to the CNS in patients in whom a brain tumour is suspected including the following are observed:
  - Progressive neurological deficit
  - New-onset seizures
  - Mental changes
  - Cranial nerve palsy
  - Unilateral sensorineural deafness
- Suspected recent-onset seizures (refer to neurologist).

Refer urgently to appropriate specialist: Patients previously diagnosed with any cancer who develop any of the following symptoms:
- Recent-onset seizure
- Progressive neurological deficit
- New mental or cognitive changes
- New neurological signs.

Consider urgent referral: Urgent referral in any patient with rapid progression of:
- Subacute focal neurological deficit
- Unexplained cognitive impairment, behavioural disturbance or slowness, or a combination of these
- Personality changes confirmed by a witness and for which there is no reasonable explanation even in the absence of the other symptoms and signs of a brain tumour.

Mouth symptoms: 📖 p.40

Hoarseness: Refer urgently for CXR if hoarseness persisting >3wk—particularly if smoker aged >50y and/or heavy drinker.

If there is a POSITIVE finding on CXR: Refer urgently to a team specializing in the management of lung cancer.

If there is a NEGATIVE finding on CXR: Refer urgently to a team specializing in the management of head and neck cancer.

Thyroid swellings:

Refer immediately to a thyroid surgeon: Patients with symptoms of tracheal compression including stridor due to thyroid swelling.

Refer urgently to a thyroid surgeon: Patients with a thyroid swelling associated with any of the following:
- Solitary nodule increasing in size
- History of neck irradiation
- Family history of an endocrine tumour
- Unexplained hoarseness or voice changes
- Cervical lymphadenopathy
- Very young (pre-pubertal) patient
- Patient aged ≥65y.

Investigation of patients who do not require urgent referral: Request TFTs in patients with a thyroid swelling without stridor or any of the features listed above.

Primary care initiation of investigations such as ultrasonography or isotope scanning is not recommended.

Refer non-urgently to endocrinology: Patients with hyper- or hypothyroidism and an associated goitre.

Refer non-urgently to a thyroid surgeon: Patients with goitre and normal thyroid function tests without any of the features listed above.

Other head and neck symptoms/signs:
Refer urgently to suitable specialist:
- Unexplained lump in the neck of recent onset
- Previously undiagnosed lump that has changed over a period of 3–6wk
- Unexplained persistent swelling in the parotid or submandibular gland
- Unexplained persistent sore or painful throat
- Unilateral unexplained pain in the head and neck area for >4wk associated with ear ache but a normal otoscopy.

Further information:
NICE Referral guidelines for suspected cancer—quick reference guide (2005) ▣ www.nice.org.uk

Suspected gastrointestinal cancer

Mouth symptoms:

Refer urgently to oral surgery: If the patient has
- Mouth ulcer(s) persisting for >3wk
- Lumps in the mouth persisting >3wk
- Red or white patches in the mouth—including suspected lichen planus—that are painful, swollen, or bleeding.

🛈 For patients with persistent symptoms/signs related to the oral cavity in whom a definitive diagnosis of a benign lesion cannot be made, refer or follow-up until the symptoms and signs disappear. If the symptoms/signs have not disappeared in ≤6wk, make an urgent referral.

Refer urgently to a dentist: Any patient with unexplained tooth mobility lasting >3wk.

Refer non-urgently to oral surgery: Patients with unexplained red and/or white patches of the oral mucosa that are not painful, swollen, or bleeding—including suspected lichen planus.

Refer to a dentist for routine monitoring: All patients with confirmed oral lichen planus

Upper GI symptoms: Consider checking FBC when referring, depending on local protocols.

Refer urgently to a team specializing in upper GI malignancy: Patients presenting with:
- Dysphagia
- Unexplained upper abdominal pain and weight ↓ ± back pain
- Upper abdominal mass without dyspepsia
- Obstructive jaundice (depending on clinical state)—consider urgent USS if available or admission to hospital.

Consider urgent referral to a specialist in upper GI malignancy: Patients presenting with:
- Persistent vomiting and weight ↓ in the absence of dyspepsia
- Unexplained weight ↓ or iron deficiency in the absence of dyspepsia
- Unexplained worsening of dyspepsia and:
  - Barrett oesophagus
  - Known dysplasia, atrophic gastritis or intestinal metaplasia
  - Peptic ulcer surgery >20y ago

Consider urgent referral to a specialist or referral for urgent endoscopy: Patients of any age with dyspepsia and:
- Chronic GI bleeding
- Dysphagia
- Progressive unintentional weight ↓
- Persistent vomiting
- Iron deficiency anaemia
- Epigastric mass
- Suspicious barium meal result.

Urgent referral for endoscopy: Any patient ≥55y and with unexplained (no obvious cause e.g. NSAIDs) and persistent, recent-onset dyspepsia alone. GPs should not allow symptoms to persist >4–6wk before referral.

① *Helicobacter pylori* status should not affect the decision to refer for suspected cancer. Consider checking a FBC to exclude iron deficiency anaemia in all patients presenting with new-onset dyspepsia.

Lower GI symptoms: Refer urgently to a team specializing in GI malignancy if:

Any age: Patient with
• Right lower abdominal mass consistent with involvement of large bowel
• A palpable rectal mass (intra-luminal, not pelvic; a pelvic mass outside the bowel would warrant an urgent referral to an urologist or gynaecologist)
• Unexplained iron deficiency anaemia (Hb ≤11 g/dl for ♂; 10 g/dl for a non-menstruating ♀).

Aged ≥40y: Reporting rectal bleeding with a change of bowel habit towards looser stools and/or increased stool frequency persisting ≥6wk.

Aged ≥60y: Patient with
• Rectal bleeding persisting for ≥6wk without a change in bowel habit and without anal symptoms
• Change in bowel habit to looser stools and/or more frequent stools persisting for ≥6wk without rectal bleeding.

① In a patient with equivocal symptoms who is not unduly anxious, it is reasonable to 'treat, watch and wait'.

Further information:
NICE Referral guidelines for suspected cancer—quick reference guide (2005) 🖥 www.nice.org.uk
SIGN Management of colorectal cancer (2003) 🖥 www.sign.ac.uk

Suspected women's cancers

Breast disease: Encourage all female patients to be breast aware. Refer any patient who presents with symptoms suggestive of breast cancer urgently (to be seen in <2wk) to a team specializing in the management of breast cancer.

Urgent referral is always required for:
Lump:
- Any age with a discrete, hard lump with fixation ± skin tethering
- Any age with a past history of breast cancer presenting with a further lump or other suspicious symptoms
- Aged ≥30y with a discrete lump that persists after the next period, or presents after menopause
- Aged <30y
  - With a lump that enlarges
  - With a lump that is fixed and hard
  - In whom there are other reasons for concern such as family history.

Nipple changes:
- Unilateral eczematous skin or nipple change that does not respond to topical treatment
- Nipple distortion of recent onset
- Spontaneous unilateral bloody nipple discharge.

Consider a non-urgent referral if:
- Woman is aged <30y and has a lump which has no suspicious features and is not enlarging
- Breast pain and no palpable abnormality, when initial treatment fails and/or symptoms persist (use of mammography is not recommended)

⚠ In patients presenting with symptoms and/or signs suggestive of breast cancer, investigation before referral is not recommended.

Abnormal vaginal bleeding: Perform a full pelvic examination, including speculum examination of the cervix, for patients with:
- Alterations in the menstrual cycle
- Inter-menstrual bleeding
- Post-coital bleeding
- Post-menopausal bleeding
- Vaginal discharge

Refer urgently to a team specializing in gynaecological cancer:
- Patients with clinical features of cervical cancer on examination. A smear test is NOT required before referral and a previous negative result should not delay referral
- All patients with post-menopausal bleeding who are NOT taking HRT
- Patients on HRT with persistent or unexplained post-menopausal bleeding after cessation of HRT for 6wk
- All patients taking tamoxifen with post-menopausal bleeding.

🛈 Endometrial thickness >4mm on USS needs further investigation.

Consider urgent referral: If persistent inter-menstrual bleeding and negative pelvic examination.

Pelvic or abdominal mass: Refer urgently for an USS if palpable abdominal or pelvic mass that is not obviously uterine fibroids or not of gastrointestinal or urological origin is found on examination. If the scan is suggestive of cancer, an urgent referral should be made. If urgent USS is not available, an urgent referral should be made.

Vulval symptoms:
Refer urgently to a team specializing in gynaecological cancer:
- Patients with an unexplained vulval lump
- Patients with vulval bleeding due to ulceration.

For patients with vulval pruritus or pain: A period of 'treat, watch and wait' is reasonable. Active follow-up is recommended until symptoms resolve or a diagnosis is confirmed. If symptoms persist, refer to gynaecology. The referral may be urgent or non-urgent, depending on the symptoms and the degree of concern about cancer.

Further information:
NICE Referral guidelines for suspected cancer—quick reference guide (2005) ▣ www.nice.org.uk
SIGN Investigation of post-menopausal bleeding (2009) ▣ www.sign.ac.uk

---

GP notes

Ovarian cancer: Ovarian cancer is notoriously difficult to diagnose. In patients with vague, non-specific, unexplained abdominal symptoms such as:
- Bloating
- Constipation
- Abdominal pain
- Back pain
- Urinary symptoms

Carry out an abdominal palpation. Also consider a pelvic examination.

Suspected urological cancer

Abdominal/pelvic mass: Refer urgently to a team specializing in urological cancer any patient with an abdominal mass identified clinically or on imaging that is thought to arise from the urinary tract.

Haematuria:

Urgent referral to a team specializing in urological cancer: Patients:
- Of any age with painless macroscopic haematuria
- Aged ≥40y with recurrent/persistent UTI associated with haematuria
- Aged ≥50y with unexplained microscopic haematuria.

Non-urgent referral: Patients <50y with microscopic haematuria. If proteinuria, ↑ serum creatinine, or ↓ eGFR, refer to a renal physician. Otherwise refer to urology.

⚠ In male patients with symptoms suggestive of UTI and macroscopic haematuria, diagnose and treat the infection before considering referral. If infection is not confirmed, refer urgently.

Prostatic symptoms/abnormal PSA: A DRE and a PSA test (after counselling) are recommended for patients with any of the following unexplained symptoms:
- Inflammatory or obstructive lower urinary tract symptoms
- Erectile dysfunction
- Haematuria
- Lower back pain
- Bone pain
- Weight loss, especially in the elderly.

Exclude UTI before PSA testing and postpone DRE until after the PSA test is done.

Interpretation of PSA results: Table 2.6, 📖 p.33

Urgent referral to a team specializing in urological cancer:
- Rectal examination—hard, irregular prostate typical of prostate cancer. PSA result should accompany the referral
- Rectal examination—normal prostate, but rising/raised age-specific PSA ± lower urinary tract symptoms*
- Symptoms and high-PSA levels
- For asymptomatic men with borderline, age-specific PSA results, repeat the PSA test after 1–3mo. If the PSA level is rising, refer the patient urgently.

*Consider discussion with specialist and patient (and/or carer) before referral for very elderly patients or those compromised by other comorbidities.

⚠ Referral is not needed if the prostate is simply enlarged and the PSA is in the age-specific reference range.

Testicular or scrotal mass:

- Refer urgently to a team specializing in urological cancer, patients with a swelling or mass in the body of the testis
- Consider an urgent USS in men with a scrotal mass that does not transilluminate and/or when the body of the testis cannot be distinguished.

Penile ulceration/masses: Refer urgently to a team specializing in management of urological cancer, all patients with symptoms or signs of penile cancer. These include the following:

- Progressive ulceration in the glans, prepuce, or skin of the penile shaft
- Mass in the glans, prepuce, or skin of the penile shaft.

❗ Lumps within the corpora cavernosa can indicate Peyronie's disease, which does not require urgent referral.

Further information:

NICE Referral guidelines for suspected cancer—quick reference guide (2005) 🖳 www.nice.org.uk

Alarm symptoms for other cancers

Suspected lung cancer:

Immediate referral/acute admission:

- Stridor
- Superior vena cava obstruction (swelling of face/neck with fixed ↑ jugular venous pressure).

Urgent referral: Refer to a team specializing in management of lung cancer:

- Persistent haemoptysis (in smokers/ex-smokers aged ≥40y)
- CXR suggestive of lung cancer (including pleural effusion and slowly resolving consolidation)
- Normal CXR where there is high suspicion of lung cancer
- History of asbestos exposure and recent onset of chest pain, shortness of breath or unexplained systemic symptoms where a CXR indicates pleural effusion, pleural mass or any suspicious lung pathology.

Urgent referral for CXR:

- Heamoptysis
- Any of the following if unexplained or present for more >3wk*:
  - Cough
  - Chest/shoulder pain
  - Dyspnoea
  - Weight loss
  - Chest signs
  - Hoarseness (refer urgently to ENT if CXR is normal)
  - Finger clubbing
  - Cervical or supraclavicular lymphadenopathy
  - Features suggestive of metastases from a lung cancer e.g. secondaries in the brain, bone, liver, or skin.

* Do not delay for 3wk if high risk of lung cancer i.e. smoker/ex-smoker, COPD, history of asbestos exposure, previous history of cancer (especially head/neck and upper GI cancer).

Suspected skin cancer:

Urgent referral: Refer patients to a team specializing in treatment of skin cancer if:

- Skin lesion suspected to be melanoma (avoid excision in primary care)
- Non-healing keratinizing or crusted skin tumour >1 cm diameter with significant induration on palpation and documented expansion over 8wk. Commonly found on the face, scalp or back of the hand
- The patient has had an organ transplant and develops a new or growing cutaneous lesion. 🛈 Squamous cell carcinoma is common with immunosuppression but may be atypical and aggressive
- Histological diagnosis of a squamous cell carcinoma.

Routine referral:

- Suspected basal cell carcinoma (usually on the face, and without significant expansion over 2mo)
- Histological diagnosis of basal cell carcinoma
- Persistent or slowly evolving unresponsive skin conditions with uncertain diagnosis.

GP notes

The 7-point check list for moles: Score 2 points for any major feature and 1 point for any minor feature. Any lesion scoring ≥3 points is suspicious—refer for consideration of skin biopsy.

Major signs:
- Change in size—increase in size
- Irregular colour
- Irregular shape—irregular border, asymmetry, elevation.

Minor signs:
- ≥7mm diameter
- Inflammation
- Oozing—including crusting or bleeding
- Change in sensation—including symptoms of minor irritation or itch.

⊙ One feature is enough to prompt referral if high level of suspicion. For low-suspicion lesions, low monitor for change over 8wk.

Minor surgery for skin lesions:
- All pigmented lesions that are not viewed as suspicious of melanoma but are excised should have a lateral excision margin of 2mm of clinically normal skin and be deep enough to include subcutaneous fat
- Send all excised skin specimens for pathological examination
- When referring a patient in whom an excised lesion has been diagnosed as malignant, send a copy of the pathology report with the referral correspondence.

Suspected bone cancer/sarcoma:

Refer for immediate X-ray: Refer for immediate X-ray any patient with suspected spontaneous pathological fracture. If the X-ray:
- Indicates possible bone cancer, refer urgently
- Is normal but symptoms persist, follow-up and/or request repeat X-ray, bone profile blood tests or referral.

Refer urgently: Refer to a team specializing in treatment of bone cancer/sarcoma if a patient presents with a palpable lump that is:
- >5 cm in diameter
- Deep to fascia, fixed, or immobile
- A recurrence after previous excision.
- Increasing in size
- Painful

If a patient has HIV consider Kaposi's sarcoma and make an urgent referral if suspected.

Urgently investigate: Increasing, unexplained, or persistent bone pain or tenderness, particularly pain at rest (and especially if not in the joint), or an unexplained limp. In older people metastases, myeloma, or lymphoma, as well as sarcoma, should be considered

Suspected haematological malignancy: This condition may present with non-specific symptoms/signs. Have a high level of suspicion.

Immediate referral:
- FBC/blood film reported as acute leukaemia
- Suspected spinal cord compression
- Suspected renal failure due to myeloma.

Urgent referral to a team specializing in blood cancers: Persistent, unexplained splenomegaly.

Investigations: Combinations of the following symptoms/signs warrant examination and further investigation with FBC, blood film, and ESR (or CRP/plasma viscosity) ± referral to a team specializing in haematological malignancy:
- Drenching night sweats and/or fever
- Weight loss
- Generalized itching—in addition check U&E, Cr, eGFR, TFTs
- Breathlessness—in addition check CXR
- Unexplained bleeding/bruising/purpura and/or symptoms suggesting anaemia
- Recurrent infections
- Persistent bone pain—in addition check X-ray, U&E, Cr and eGFR, liver profile, bone profile, and PSA (in men)
- Alcohol-induced pain
- Abdominal pain
- Splenomegaly—refer if persistent

- Fatigue—Repeat FBC, blood film, and ESR or CRP at least once if condition remains unexplained and does not improve
- Lymphadenopathy—if present ≥6wk, LNs are increasing in size, LN >2cm in size, widespread lymphadenopathy, or associated weight ↓ night sweats and/or splenomegaly, consider further investigation, discussion with specialist and/or referral.

Further information:

NICE Referral guidelines for suspected cancer—quick reference guide (2005) ▣ www.nice.org.uk

Diagnosis of cancer in children

Diagnosis of childhood malignancy is a particular challenge in primary care. GPs rarely see children affected with cancer and the cancers that affect children are often unfamiliar to them. Always have a high index of suspicion and, if in doubt, refer for a specialist opinion. Referrals should be made to a paediatrician or specialist in children's cancer.

⚠ Some congenital/genetic syndromes may be associated with ↑ risk of childhood cancer (e.g. Down's syndrome—leukaemia; neurofibromatosis—CNS tumours).

Investigations: Check FBC and blood film if:
- Pallor and/or fatigue
- Unexplained irritability
- Unexplained fever
- Persistent or recurrent UTIs
- Generalized lymphadenopathy
- Persistent or unexplained bone pain (additionally consider X-ray)
- Unexplained bruising.

⚠ If the blood film or FBC indicates leukaemia, make an *urgent referral*.

Abdominal distension: If persistent or progressive, examine the abdomen:
- If a mass is found, refer immediately
- If the child is uncooperative and abdominal examination is not possible or if examination is difficult, consider referral for urgent abdominal USS.

Immediate referral/admission: Any child with:
- Hepatosplenomegaly
- Unexplained petechiae
- Unexplained urinary retention
- ↓ conscious level
- Headache and vomiting that cause early morning waking or occur on waking as these are classic signs of ↑ intra-cranial pressure ⚠ <1% of patients presenting with headache have a brain tumour
- Children <2y with new-onset seizures (excluding febrile convulsion); bulging fontanelle; extensor attacks; and/or persistent vomiting
- Mediastinal, hilar, or thoracic mass on CXR.

Urgent/immediate referral: Any child with:
- New-onset seizures
- Cranial nerve abnormalities
- Visual disturbances
- Leg weakness—refer immediately if gait abnormalities or motor or sensory signs
- Other motor/sensory signs
- Abdominal mass
- Skin nodules in a baby which could be metastatic neuroblastoma
- Proptosis
- Shortness of breath—particularly if not responding to bronchodilators
- FBC suggesting malignancy.

Urgent referral: Urgently refer

- When a child presents several times (≥3×) with the same problem, but with no clear diagnosis
- If white papillary reflex (leukocoria)—Figure 3.1.
- If aged ≥2y with persistent headache where you cannot carry out an adequate neurological examination in primary care
- If aged <2y with:
  - Abnormal ↑ in head size
  - Arrest/regression of motor development and/or altered behaviour
  - Abnormal eye movements and/or lack of visual following
  - Poor feeding/failure to thrive
  - New squint/change in visual acuity—urgency depends on other factors.
- If unexplained mass at any site that has ≥1 of the following features— the mass is:
  - Deep to the fascia
  - Non-tender
  - Progressively enlarging
  - Associated with a regional LN that is enlarging
  - >2cm in diameter in size.
- If lymphadenopathy with ≥1 of the following features (particularly if no evidence of local infection and/or associated with general ill health, fever, or weight loss):
  - Non-tender, firm, or hard LNs
  - Lymph nodes >2cm in size
  - Lymph nodes progressively enlarging
  - Any axillary nodes (in the absence of local infection or dermatitis)
  - Any supraclavicular nodes.
- If haematuria
- If persistent localized bone pain/swelling and X-ray showing signs of cancer
- If unexplained deteriorating school performance or developmental milestones, or unexplained behavioural and/or mood changes
- If rest pain or unexplained limp—consider X-ray and/or discussion with a paediatrician before or as well as referral
- If family history of retinoblastoma and visual problems.

Unexplained or persistent back pain: Examine the child and check FBC and blood film. Consider X-ray and/or discussion with a paediatrician. If no cause is found, *refer urgently.*

Consider referral: When there is persistent parental anxiety, even when a benign cause is considered most likely.

Figure 3.1 White papillary reflex in a child with retinoblastoma

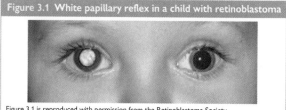

Figure 3.1 is reproduced with permission from the Retinoblastoma Society.

Chapter 4

Principles of cancer treatment

Treatment decisions

If cancer is suspected, as a result of signs or symptoms locally at the original site or at distant sites, an accurate and comprehensive assessment of both the patient and the disease must be undertaken before a treatment decision is reached.

Assessment of the tumour:

Histological nature of the tumour: Tumour specimens, usually obtained through fine-needle biopsy, core biopsy, surgical biopsy, or excision of a mass or lesion, are examined to confirm:

- Malignancy
- The tissue in which the cancer originated
- If the cancer has been fully excised
- The histopathological type e.g. adenocarcinoma, squamous carcinoma
- The degree of differentiation e.g. well, moderately, or poorly differentiated
- The tumour grade e.g. low, intermediate, or high grade

High grade, poorly differentiated tumours tend to have a poorer outcome than low-grade, well-differentiated tumours.

Biological behaviour of the tumour: Tumour markers produced by cancers may be a useful adjunct to histological classification and staging and can be used to influence and monitor efficacy of treatment—Table 4.1. ⓘ tumour markers can be ↑ in many non-malignant conditions.

Anatomical extent of the tumour: Usually determined through a combination of clinical, radiological (Table 4.2), biochemical and surgical assessment. Routine blood tests including liver function tests and bone profiles may also indicate the presence of metastases.

Cancer staging

Once assessment has been completed the stage of the tumour should be determined. Staging aims to:

- Allow the clinician to determine the aim of treatment (palliative or curative)
- Aid the clinician in planning the type of treatment
- Give some indication of prognosis for the patient
- Evaluate the efficacy of treatment by repeating investigations following therapy.

The TMN classification: This is a widely used classification of tumours. Exact criteria for staging depend on the primary organ site:

- T—Primary tumour—graded T_1–T_4 with increasing size of primary
- N—Regional lymph nodes—advancing nodal disease is graded N_0–N_3
- M—Presence (M_1) or absence (M_0) of metastases.

Stage grouping:

- *Stage 1:* Clinical examination reveals a tumour confined to the primary organ. The lesion tends to be operable and completely resectable
- *Stage 2:* Clinical examination shows evidence of local spread into surrounding tissue and first draining lymph nodes. The lesion is also operable and resectable but there is a higher risk of further spread of the disease
- *Stage 3:* Clinical examination reveals an extensive primary tumour with fixation to deeper structures and local invasion. The lesion may not be operable and may require a combination of treatment modalities
- *Stage 4:* Evidence of distant metastases beyond the site of origin. The primary site may be surgically inoperable.

Table 4.1 Tumour markers and associated conditions

Tumour marker	Associated conditions	
	Malignant conditions	**Non-malignant conditions**
CEA	GI tract cancers (particularly colorectal cancer)	Cirrhosis Pancreatitis Smoking Inflammation
CA 19–9	Colorectal cancer Pancreatic cancer	Cholestasis Obstructive jaundice
CA 125	Ovarian cancer Breast cancer Hepatocellular cancer	Cirrhosis Pregnancy Peritonitis
α FP	Hepatocellular cancer Germ cell cancers (not pure seminoma)	Cirrhosis Pregnancy Hepatitis Open neural tube defects
HCG	Germ cell cancers Choriocarcinoma and hydatidiform mole	Pregnancy
PSA	Prostate cancer	Benign prostatic hypertrophy Prostatitis Prostate instrumentation (including rectal examination) Acute urinary retention Physical exercise Old age

Table 4.2 Features of gastric and duo-denal ulcers

Imaging technique	Preferred when evaluating
CT	Lungs, abdominal cavity
Spiral CT	Makes 3-D images of areas inside the body. Detects small abnormal areas better than conventional CT.
MRI	Mediastinum, liver, pelvis, brain, spinal cord
PET	By using FDG (radio-labelled glucose) which is avidly taken up by actively dividing cells, helps to: Determine functional and metabolic status of tumours Distinguish benign from malignant lesions Distinguish whether a residual mass after treatment represents fibrosis or residual tumour.

Advice for patients

Further information about treatment decisions:

- Cancer Research UK ☎ 0808 800 4040 🖥 www.cancerhelp.org.uk
- Macmillan Cancer Support ☎ 0808 800 0000
  🖥 www.macmillar.org.uk
- Patient experience database 🖥 www.healthtalkonline.org

Patient's performance status: To predict which patients are likely to benefit from oncological interventions, oncologists rely on the patient's functional status—the Eastern Co-operative Oncology Group (ECOG) Performance Status Scale is widely used (Table 4.3).

Mortality, morbidity, and efficacy: These factors will be considered by the consultant oncologist when deciding on treatment. The GP may be contacted by the patient to help explain the risks and benefits of treatments offered, or if given a choice of treatment options by the consultant. In such circumstances maintaining open communication with the oncology team and availing of up-to-date literature may help.

Patient preferences: Before any treatment decision is reached the preferences of the patient should be sought and discussed.

Clinical trials: Clinical research is essential to advance medical knowledge and improve patient outcome. Many patients diagnosed with cancer will be offered the opportunity of participating in a clinical trial to determine whether new therapies are more effective or have less side effects than standard care and/or the best method of treatment (Table 4.4). In general, patients participating in clinical trials do *better* than patients receiving standard treatment, but before agreeing to participate in any trial, patients should take time to:

- Ensure that they read all the information provided about the trial
- Ask for further explanation if they do not understand anything or if further information is needed
- Weigh the risks and additional inconveniences against the benefits of taking part in a trial.

End points of clinical trials: Common end points include:

- Disease-free survival (in adjuvant studies)
- Overall survival (in palliative studies)
- Health economics (costs versus effects)
- Time to progression
- Response
- Toxicity
- Quality of life
- Health economics.

Further information:

Watson et al. *Oncology—Oxford Core Text* (2nd edition—2006) OUP ISBN: 13: 9780198567578

Adjuvant online—decision making tool for professionals. assessing risks and benefits of additional therapy after surgery ▣ www.adjuvantonline.com

Table 4.3 Eastern Co-operative Oncology Group (ECOG) performance status scale

Classification	Description
ECOG 0	Fully active; able to carry on all activities without restriction.
ECOG 1	Restricted in physically strenuous activity but ambulatory and able to carry out work of a light or sedentary nature.
ECOG 2	Ambulatory and capable of all self-care; confined to bed or chair 50% of waking hours.
ECOG 3	Capable of only limited self-care; confined to bed or chair 50% or more of waking hours.
ECOG 4	Completely disabled; cannot carry on any self-care; totally confined to bed or chair.

ⓘ Patients with ECOG score >2 are usually deemed unsuitable for most chemotherapy interventions.

Table 4.4 Clinical trial stages

Trial phase	Aims to	Eligible patients
I	Establish the human toxicity of a new drug through delivering carefully selected increasing doses to patients. Establish a safe dose and schedule at which to start further trials with the drug. Evaluate the body's handling of the drug by pharmacokinetic studies and effects of drug on tumour or normal tissues by pharmacodynamic studies.	Patients with progressive disease despite standard oncological therapy or with tumours for which no standard therapy exists. Patients must be aware that the primary objective is to assess tolerability and side effects and that there is little expectation of benefit for themselves, with a historical response rate of 5%. Patients must have a good performance status and are usually highly motivated as involvement often involves frequent hospital visits and investigations. Usually small numbers of patients are involved e.g. 10–40.
II	Establish the anti-tumour activity of a drug for a particular tumour type.	Patients with progressive disease despite standard oncological therapy or with tumours for which no standard therapy exists. Patients usually have a good performance status and motivation. Patients are closely monitored with toxicity and response assessments but not as intensively as those in Phase I studies. Usually moderate numbers of patients are involved e.g. 50–300.
III	Compare the new drug or combination with conventional therapy.	Patients for whom a standard therapy exists—new drugs may also be compared with 'best supportive care' where no standard therapy exists. Usually large numbers of patients are involved e.g. several hundreds to many thousands.

Treatment intent

The goals of cancer treatment should be clearly defined. Cancer treatment can be:

Radical

- Treatment with curative intent, involving surgery, radiotherapy, chemotherapy in isolation or combination
- As this is treatment with curative intent a relatively high incidence of treatment toxicity is acceptable
- Good symptom control and psychological support is essential to encourage completion of very demanding treatments—without this the patient may miss their only opportunity of cure
- Long-term side effects from cumulative dose toxicities should be considered and minimized, e.g. cardiotoxicities from anthracyclines.

Adjuvant

- Treatment given after surgery when no evidence of metastatic disease present but occult micro-metastatic disease known to be possible
- Shown to improve long-term survival in patients with micro-metastatic disease not clinically apparent at the time of primary treatment e.g. breast and colonic cancer
- Few predictive factors to identify those who will benefit from adjuvant therapy
- Decision to proceed is based on the likelihood of relapse
- As most patients will not benefit acute toxicity should be manageable and have a low risk of long-term complications.

Palliative

- Treatment indicated when cure is not possible
- May improve quality of life and cancer-related symptoms
- Can delay progression of disease and prolong survival
- May involve clinically detectable tumour shrinkage but palliative benefit has been shown to be obtained even in the absence of such shrinkage
- Treatment should usually be well tolerated with a low incidence of acute side effects—an exception may be patients receiving primary chemotherapy for an advanced but chemosensitive tumour e.g. advanced ovarian cancer
- Long-term toxicities are generally not relevant.

GP notes

Adjusting to different treatment goals: The switch to palliative treatment with fewer investigations and change in emphasis to symptomatic management can be very difficult for patients and carers who have experienced radical and adjuvant therapy, often evoking feelings of abandonment. These patients in particular may need additional support from their primary care team.

The GP's role in cancer care: Treatment for cancer is increasingly successful but also increasingly complex. GPs often feel bewildered by the investigations ordered and treatments given and cannot hope to stay up-to-date with current thinking on treatment of every kind of cancer. Although treatment of cancer is largely a specialist activity, the role of the GP is important at this time, even if it is peripheral:

- Keep in touch with the family and up-to-date with what is going on
- Provide support to the patient and other family members
- Provide general medical care, referring back to oncology or palliative care promptly as needed
- Provide preventative care e.g. flu vaccination for patients and/or carers
- Ensure prescriptions requested by specialist services are supplied promptly
- Co-ordinate care with other members of the primary care team and/or other services
- Provide continuity when care is passed from one secondary care team to another
- Give advice on any benefits or local services the family might find of assistance
- If the patient does not survive, provide ongoing support to family members after the patient has died.

Surgery

Surgery has three main roles in cancer management:

Diagnosis and staging: Advances in diagnostic imaging and interventional radiology, endoscopy, and laparoscopic techniques have dramatically reduced the number of patients requiring open surgery to confirm a cancer diagnosis. However, surgical staging remains important in:

- Breast cancer—'sentinel' axillary node biopsy is needed to accurately predict the state of nodal disease
- Ovarian cancer—tumour deposits on the peritoneal surface are poorly visualized with conventional imaging. Direct visualization is required using laparotomy or laparoscopy
- Certain abdominal malignancies—laparoscopic assessment of the extent and spread of tumour is performed before major resection e.g. gastroesophageal cancer.

Curative surgery

Non-metastatic disease: Surgery with curative intent is dependent on complete resection of the tumour with a margin of normal tissue. Local control of tumours with a propensity to spread to lymph nodes may be improved with resection of the draining group of nodes e.g. vulval tumours. However, even if the tumour was completely resected, surgery can still fail to cure either as a result of:

- Development of metastatic disease as a result of the presence of micro-metastatic deposits unidentifiable at the time of surgery
- Development of local relapse as a result of inadequate margins. Surgical margins can be limited by patient-related factors (e.g. only a partial lobectomy may be possible in patients with lung cancer because of poor underlying respiratory function) or by tumour-related margins (e.g. invasion of the tumour of a vital structure such as the aorta).

Metastatic disease: Surgery may be curative in a limited number of tumours with metastases. However, this is much less common, requires careful patient selection, thorough re-staging, careful patient counselling and is best performed by a specialist team. Circumstances in which curative surgery may be offered include the following:

- Isolated brain metastases from breast, renal cell, and colorectal cancer with a long disease-free interval
- Liver metastases from colorectal cancer
- Pulmonary metastases from osteosarcoma, soft tissue sarcoma, testicular tumours, or colorectal cancer.

Palliative surgery: Surgery can be effective in achieving good symptom control in the palliative setting, but decision to proceed must be carefully considered particularly as patients may have limited life expectancy, poor performance status, and rapid tumour progression. Ideally such decisions should be multi-disciplinary and involve surgeons specialized in oncology and experienced in palliative management. See Table 4.5.

Further information:

Cassidy et al. Oxford Handbook of Oncology (2nd edition—2006) OUP ISBN: 0198567871
Watson et al. Oncology—Oxford Core Text (2nd edition—2006) OUP ISBN: 13: 9780198567578

Table 4.5 Situations in which palliative surgery or other interventional procedures should be considered

Situation	Comments
Cancers causing obstructive symptoms e.g. bowel, ovary, ureter, bronchus	Surgery to relieve the obstruction may be warranted even if the underlying disease is incurable with locally advanced disease or distant metastases. *Bowel obstruction*—this occurs most commonly in patients with colonic or ovarian cancer. *Oesophageal or bronchial obstruction*—laser therapy of an intra-luminal mass may restore the lumen. *Obstructive hydronephrosis*—nephrostomy or ureteric catheters may relieve the obstruction. *Placement of a stent*—may help relieve the symptoms of dysphagia, dyspnoea, jaundice, and large bowel obstruction.
Fistulae	Fistulae, often arising as a result of uncontrolled pelvic tumours or as a side effect of radiotherapy, can be associated with distressing malodours and excessive discharge. Surgery may provide excellent palliation but may not be useful in those with multiple sites of fistulae or rapidly advancing intra-abdominal disease where life expectancy is limited.
Jaundice	Radiological and/or endoscopic stent placement—can relieve obstructive jaundice secondary to extrinsic pressure from lymph nodes on the biliary system or intrinsic pressure from cholangiocarcinoma or pancreatic carcinoma. *Complications*—infection or blockage necessitate replacement. *Surgical relief*—by choledochoenterostomy, avoids the problems associated with stents and may be indicated in a small minority with excellent performance status and slowly growing disease.
Spinal cord compression and brain tumours	Urgent referral for neurological assessment for decompressive surgery is indicated for confirmed spinal disease or operable brain tumours.
Gastrointestinal bleeding	A wide range of endoscopic techniques have been developed to stop bleeding from benign and malignant causes including sclerotherapy with adrenaline, laser coagulation, and radiological embolization. These techniques may avoid the need for major surgery in patients who have a limited life expectancy.
Bone metastases	Prophylactic fixation of a long bone may reduce either pain and/or the risk of pathological fracture in patients with • Lesions in weight bearing bones • Destruction of >50% of the cortex • Pain on weight bearing • Lytic lesions. In all cases fixation should be followed by radiotherapy to control growth and promote healing.
Pain	If the expected morbidity of the procedure is low, surgical debulking of large, slowly growing tumours can reduce pain. Neurosurgical approaches such as cordotomy are only rarely considered. Destructive techniques such as radiofrequency ablation performed percutaneously or laparoscopically have an increasing role in palliating symptoms from expanding primary or secondary tumour masses.

Radiotherapy

Radiotherapy is widely used in the treatment of patients with cancer, both in curative and palliative settings

Mechanism of action: Ionizing radiation damages cells. Radiotherapy aims to deliver a dose of irradiation to an area that allows normal tissues, but not the cancer, to recover from the damage.

Delivery of radiotherapy: Radiotherapy may be used alone or with chemotherapy. Once maximum dose of radiotherapy has been received by any area that area cannot usually be irradiated again.

External beam: An external source of ionizing radiation (e.g. gamma rays) is aimed at a target point in the body. Patients may be immobilized e.g. with special boards/moulds, to ensure delivery of treatment to the correct place. Can be single dose (e.g. for palliative reasons) or fractionated into several doses spread over weeks e.g. 25 fractions over 5wk. Fractionation ↑ effect.

Brachytherapy: Delivery of radiation by placing a radioactive source within or close to the malignancy e.g. caesium^{137} placed in the uterus or Iodine or Iridium in the prostate.

Curative treatment: Radiotherapy may be used for curative treatment in preference to, or as an alternative to surgical treatment for: lymphoma; seminoma; childhood tumours (medulloblastoma, neuroblastoma, Wilm tumour); head/neck tumours; early cervical cancer; bladder cancer; squamous/basal cell skin cancer; anal cancer (with chemotherapy); non-small cell lung cancer (if unfit for surgery).

Adjuvant radiotherapy: Used pre-operatively to ↓ size/extent of otherwise inoperable tumours, or post-operatively to treat microscopic foci or potential micrometastases remaining after tumour removal (e.g. in treatment of breast cancer).

Palliative radiotherapy: It is used to control distressing symptoms:
- Only symptomatic sites of disease are targeted
- Single dose/short fractionation regimens are used
- Palliative benefit must outweigh treatment-related toxicity

Examples:
- *Pain*—bone metastases, nerve compression, and soft tissue infiltration. If bone pain is diffuse, hemibody radiation may be effective. An alternative is IV radioisotope therapy with strontium^{89} or samarium^{153}
- *Obstruction of a viscus*—bronchial obstruction, superior vena cava obstruction due to radio-sensitive tumours, or obstruction with other tumours where stenting is not an option or a stent has overgrown
- *Haemorrhage*—Haemoptysis, haematuria, haematemesis, per vaginal bleeding, rectal bleeding
- *Neurological complications*—spinal cord compression, symptomatic brain metastases, pain from cranial or peripheral nerve compression due to breast or prostate cancer (nerve palsies seldom recover)
- *Fungating tumours*—if surgery is not possible or felt to be inappropriate, radiotherapy ↓ the tumour mass, serous ooze or haemorrhage, and may promote healing.

Common side effects of radiotherapy: See Table 4.6.

Table 4.6 Side effects of radiotherapy

Side effect	Description/action
Skin	Erythema ± desquamation—📖 p.182
Sore mouth/ throat	Associated with radiotherapy to the head/neck.
	Advice—visit the dentist before treatment; avoid smoking, alcohol, and spicy foods; rest voice when radiotherapy reaction becomes established.
	Consider treatment with—normal saline/bicarbonate mouthwashes; antiseptic mouth washes (e.g. chlorhexidine—though alcohol may sting); soluble aspirin (can be gargled) or paracetamol; benzydamine spray/mouthwash; topical local anaesthetics (e.g. xylocaine gel); topical steroids (e.g. Adcortyl® in Orabase® paste, hydrocortisone pellets); coating agents (e.g. sucralfate).
	If insufficient fluid/food intake, consider nutritional support via NG tube and/or referral for gastrostomy (if weight loss >10%).
Dysphagia	May result from thoracic radiotherapy.
	Avoid smoking, spirits, and spicy food.
	Consider treatment with—antacid (e.g. Gaviscon®); sucralfate; soluble paracetamol, or Aspirin; NSAID PO/PR.
Nausea and vomiting	Radiotherapy to the abdomen often causes nausea as a result of serotonin release. Consider prophylactic anti-emetic therapy with a serotonin inhibitor e.g. ondansetron.
Diarrhoea	Frequently accompanies abdominal/pelvic radiotherapy.
	Management: dietary modification (e.g. ↓ dietary fibre) may help. Supply with loperamide—4mg initial dose then 2mg every 2h until symptoms settle (4mg every 4h at night).
	Proctitis—may accompany rectal/prostatic irradiation. Treat with rectal steroids.
Pneumonitis	Acute pneumonitis can develop 1–3mo after treatment and is associated with a fever, dry cough, and breathlessness.
	Differential diagnosis: pneumonia.
	Investigation: CXR—shows lung infiltration confined within the treatment volume.
	Management: Steroids—start with 40mg od prednisolone and reduce over a period of weeks as improvement occurs.
	ⓘ Pulmonary fibrosis may occur >12mo after treatment.
Cerebral oedema	Can occur after cranial irradiation, especially if no surgery to the tumour. Steroid dose is ↓ after completion of radiotherapy. Consider ↑ dose again.
Somnolence syndrome	Occurs within a few weeks of brain irradiation.
	Presents with: Nausea/vomiting; anorexia; dysarthria; ataxia; profound lethargy.
	Treatment is supportive. Recovery may occur spontaneously.
Fatigue	Occurs commonly during and after irradiation. Treatment is supportive. Recovery will occur but may take time.

Chemotherapy

Chemotherapy is the use of chemical agents in the cure or palliation of malignant disease. Traditionally, these were cytotoxic agents which acted as non-specific cellular poisons. Increasingly, biological agents which are targeted specifically to tumours are being developed and used.

Drug groups: These include the following:
- Antibiotics e.g. bleomycin
- Alkylating agents e.g. busulfan
- Anti-metabolites e.g. methotrexate, 5-fluorouracil
- Alkaloids e.g. vincristine
- Platinum derivatives—DNA intercalating agents e.g. cisplatin
- Enzymes e.g. asparaginase
- Hormones e.g. sex hormones, corticosteroids
- Biological agents e.g. BCG, interferon-alfa, trastuzumab (Herceptin®), rituximab
- Others e.g. hydroxyurea, retinoids.

These agents work in a variety of ways to inhibit tumour growth and/or cause tumour cell damage. Normal cells may be damaged at the same time as tumour cells, resulting in the high levels of toxicity experienced by some patients.

Choice of agent: Choice of the systemic therapy such as cytotoxic chemotherapy depends on known activity of the agent, cost, and patient factors. It is a specialist decision.

Types of tumour: Response to chemotherapy depends on type and grade of tumour being treated. Broadly tumours can be divided into:
- *Those likely to respond*—leukaemia, lymphoma (Hodgkin and intermediate/high-grade non-Hodgkin), testicular tumours, small cell lung cancer, embryonal tumours, choriocarcinoma, ovarian cancer, sarcoma, breast cancer, prostate cancer, colorectal cancer
- *Those that may respond*—low-grade non-Hodgkin lymphoma, upper GI cancer, brain/CNS tumours, melanoma, bladder cancer, uterine cancer
- *Those unlikely to respond*—non-small cell lung cancer, renal cancer, pancreatic cancer, head and neck cancer, cervical cancer, liver cancer.

Combination chemotherapy: Often different chemotherapeutic agents are combined to increase their chances of effect. Agents acting in different ways may potentiate each others' actions and using combinations reduces the risk of resistance (if one agent does not have any effect, another may). Choosing agents with different side-effect profiles reduces cumulative toxic effects.

Intermittent chemotherapy: This is particularly useful for cytotoxic drugs. Intermittent treatment exploits the difference in recovery rates between normal and malignant tissues. Gaps between cycles of treatment allow normal tissue (particularly the bone marrow) to recover, but the malignant tissue does not recover to such a large extent (Figure 4.1, 📖 p.71). The population of malignant cells diminishes relative to the normal cells with each cycle.

Adjuvant chemotherapy: This therapy is used to prevent relapse after primary treatment of a non-metastatic tumour for which relapse rate is known to be high. A good example is adjuvant chemotherapy for breast cancer.

Specific chemotherapeutic agents: With a constantly changing array of chemotherapeutic agents it can be very hard to keep track of the key facts needed to manage patients in the community while they are receiving chemotherapy. The following list of commonly used systemic therapies has been compiled with this in mind:
- Conventional cytotoxic chemotherapeutic agents—Table 4.7
- Biological agents—Table 4.8, 🕮 p.72
- Hormone therapy—Table 4.9, 🕮 p.73.

⚠ Before stopping any chemotherapy agent, discuss with the consultant in charge of the patient's care.

Table 4.7 Indications and side effects for common cytotoxic chemotherapy agents	
Agent	**Indications and potential problems**
Bleomycin Anti-tumour antibiotic Given IV/ intra-cavity	*Used for*: germ cell tumours, lymphoma, malignant pleural effusions. *Toxicities*: commonly fever and chills within hours of administration; hyperpigmentation of skin; peeling skin on fingertips; pulmonary fibrosis (↑ risk if smoker—advise smoking cessation). *If new onset/increasing dyspnoea*: refer for CXR and pulmonary function tests.
Busulfan Alkylating agent Given IV/PO	*Used for*: leukaemia. *Toxicities*: prolonged myelosuppression (up to 30d.); bronze hyperpigmentation of the skin; pulmonary fibrosis. ❶ Concomitant itraconazole can ↑ toxicity.
Capecitabine (Xeloda®) Fluropyrimidine anti-metabolite (pro-drug of 5-FU) Given PO	*Used for*: breast cancer, GI cancer. *Toxicities*: diarrhoea; stomatitis; nausea; vomiting; *hand-foot syndrome* (palmar-plantar erythema and paraesthesia); angina, myelosuppression. ❶ Administration concurrently with warfarin can cause bleeding. Monitor INR closely or change to low-molecular weight heparin. *If severe GI toxicity*: stop treatment until symptoms resolve. Rehydration and electrolyte replacement may be needed. *If painful blistering on hands*: discontinue treatment until symptoms resolve then reduce dose. Pyridoxine (vitamin B_6) 50mg tds may help.
Carboplatin DNA intercalating agent Given IV	*Used for*: lung cancer; ovarian cancer; germ cell tumours. *Toxicities*: thrombocytopoenia (↑ risk of bleeding if taking anti-platelet medication as well); myelosuppression; nausea/vomiting; hypersensitivity reactions. Renal impairment exacerbates haematological toxicity—dose is adjusted based on renal function.
Chlorambucil Alkylating agent Given PO	*Used for*: leukaemia; lymphoma. *Toxicities*: myelosuppression; thrombocytopenia; rash (rarely progresses to Stevens-Johnson syndrome).

Table 4.7 (Contd.)

Agent	Indications and potential problems
Cisplatin DNA intercalating agent Given IV	*Used for*: lung, head and neck, bladder, uterine, upper GI, and germ cell tumours. *Toxicities*: severe nausea/vomiting (may persist up to 96h following administration); myelosuppression; metallic taste; nephrotoxicity (↑ serum Cr, hypomagnesaemia); tinnitus; peripheral neuropathy; constipation. FBC, renal function and electrolytes should be monitored throughout treatment. *If severe emesis persists*: consider anti-emetic via syringe driver, ensure adequate hydration (dehydration exacerbates nephrotoxic effects). ⓘ Avoid concomitant use of nephrotoxic or ototoxic drugs e.g. NSAIDs, aminoglycoside antibiotics, loop diuretics.
Cyclophosphamide Alkylating agent Given IV/PO	*Used for*: breast cancer, lymphoma. *Toxicities*: hair loss; myelosuppression; haemorrhagic cystitis (Mesna is given before administration as a urothelial protectant); nausea/vomiting. FBC should be monitored during treatment. ⓘ ↑ anti-coagulant effect of warfarin.
Cytarabine Anti-metabolite Given IV, SC or intra-thecally	*Used for*: leukaemia, lymphoma. *Toxicities*: myelosuppression; thrombocytopenia; anaemia; nausea/vomiting; metallic taste; diarrhoea; headache (following intra-thecal administration). FBC should be monitored during treatment.
Dacarbazine Alkylating agent Given IV	*Used for*: melanoma, lymphoma. *Toxicities*: myelosuppression; thrombocytopenia; nausea/vomiting; abnormal LFTs. FBC and LFTs should be monitored during treatment.
Daunorubicin Anthracycline anti-tumour antibiotic Given IV	*Used for*: leukaemia. *Toxicities*: as for doxorubicin

---

Advice for patients

Information about side effects of chemotherapy:

Chemocare ⌨ www.chemocare.com
Cancer Research UK ☎ 0808 800 4040 ⌨ www.cancerhelp.org.uk
Macmillan Cancer Support ☎ 0808 808 0000
⌨ www.macmillan.org.uk

Table 4.7 (Contd.)

Agent	Indications and potential problems
Docetaxel (Taxotere®) Taxane (anti-microtubule agent) Given IV	*Used for:* breast, lung, prostate, head and neck and upper GI cancers. *Toxicities:* hair loss; myelosuppression; peripheral neuropathy; arthralgia; myalgia; fluid retention; nail changes (discolouration, separation from the nail bed); hypersensitivity reactions (rash, flushing, low-back ache, anaphylactoid reactions with hypotension ± bronchospasm). Pre-medication with a 3d course of dexamethasone ↓ incidence of hypersensitivity reactions. ❶ Toxicity is ↑ in patients with abnormal LFTs. Diabetic patients with diabetic neuropathy are more susceptible to drug-induced neuropathy.
Doxorubicin (Adriamycin®) Anthracycline anti-tumour antibiotic Given IV	*Used for:* breast cancer, lymphoma, sarcoma. *Toxicities:* hair loss; myelosuppression; stomatitis; nausea/vomiting; congestive cardiac failure with cumulative exposure; exacerbation of angina or arrhythmia; skin blistering, ulceration and tissue necrosis if extravasates (vesicant); colours urine red; may cause *radiation recall reaction* (sunburn-like reaction in the area of previous radiotherapy). FBC should be monitored during treatment. *If chest pain or dyspnoea:* check ECG and refer for echo and cardiac assessment. Risk is ↑ if underlying cardiac risk factors or previous mediastinal irradiation. *If extravasation has occurred:* monitor the affected skin closely. If ulceration with tissue necrosis develops, may require referral to plastic surgery.
Liposomal doxorubicin (Caelyx®) Pegylated formulation of doxorubicin Given IV	*Used for:* breast cancer, ovarian cancer, Kaposi sarcoma. *Toxicities:* similar to doxorubicin but less cardiotoxic and non-vesicant. May also cause hand-foot syndrome (palmar-plantar erythema and paraesthesia).
Epirubicin Anthracycline anti-tumour antibiotic Given IV	*Used for:* breast cancer, upper GI malignancy. *Toxicities:* similar to doxorubicin but less cardiotoxic.
Etoposide Topoisomerase II inhibitor Given IV/PO	*Used for:* lymphoma, leukaemia, germ cell tumours, small cell lung cancer. *Toxicities:* hair loss; nausea/vomiting; myelosuppression; risk of secondary leukaemia. FBC should be monitored during treatment. ❶ ↑ anti-coagulant effect of warfarin.
Fludarabine Anti-metabolite Given IV	*Used for:* lymphoma, leukaemia. *Toxicities:* myelosuppression; thrombocytopenia; neurological symptoms (drowsiness, confusion); pneumonitis. FBC should be monitored during treatment.

Table 4.7 (*Contd.*)

Agent	Indications and potential problems
5-fluorouracil Anti-metabolite Given IV/ intra-arterially/ topically	*Used for:* colorectal cancer, upper GI cancer, skin cancer. *Toxicities:* myelosuppression; stomatitis; diarrhoea; hand-foot syndrome (palmar-plantar erythema and paraesthesia); photosensitivity; phlebitis; neurological symptoms (headache, ataxia, confusion); dry eyes; excessive lacrimation due to tear duct stenosis. ⬤ Pyridoxine (vitamin B_6) 50mg tds may alleviate symptoms of hand-foot syndrome.
Gemcitabine Anti-metabolite Given IV	*Used for:* non-small cell lung cancer; bladder cancer; pancreatic cancer; breast cancer. *Toxicities:* myelosuppression; rash; 'flu-like' symptoms; fatigue; pulmonary fibrosis; pneumonitis; radiation recall (sunburn-like reaction in area of previous radiotherapy) abnormal LFTs (↑ transaminases, ↑ bilirubin).
Hydroxycarbamide *(Hydroxyurea)* Anti-metabolite Given PO	*Used for:* leukaemia and myeloproliferative disease. *Toxicities:* myelosuppression; thrombocytopenia; anaemia; rash; renal impairment. FBC and renal function should be monitored during treatment.
Ifosfamide Alkylating agent Given IV	*Used for:* sarcoma, germ cell tumours, lung cancer. *Toxicities:* hair loss; myelosuppression; haemorrhagic cystitis (Mesna is given before administration as a uro-protectant); nausea/vomiting, neurological toxicity (drowsiness, confusion, coma—exacerbated by impaired renal function). FBC and renal function should be monitored during treatment.
Irinotecan Topoisomerase I inhibitor Given IV	*Used for:* colorectal cancer. *Toxicities:* cholinergic syndrome (lacrimation, diarrhoea, and abdominal cramps during/just after administration—severity of symptoms is ↓ by atropine pre-medication); diarrhoea (early onset associated with cholinergic syndrome, or late onset >24h after administration due to GI mucosal toxicity); myelosuppression; nausea/vomiting. *If diarrhoea develops >24h after infusion:* give loperamide 4mg at first loose stool then 2mg every 2h (4mg every 4h at night) until no diarrhoea for 12h. Consult oncology team if symptoms do not respond to loperamide within 48h or if dehydrated or unwell.
Lomustine (CCNU; *CeeNU®)* Alkylating agent (nitrosourea) Given PO	*Used for:* primary and secondary brain tumours; lymphoma. *Toxicities:* Delayed myelosuppression—reaches maximum suppression ≈6wk after administration; nausea/vomiting. FBC should be monitored during treatment.

Table 4.7 (*Contd.*)

Agent	Indications and potential problems
Melphalan Alkylating agent Given IV/PO	*Used for:* myeloma. *Toxicities:* delayed myelosuppression—reaches maximum suppression ≈4wk after administration. FBC should be monitored during treatment.
Mercaptopurine Anti-metabolite Given PO	*Used for:* leukaemia, lymphoma. *Toxicities:* myelosuppression, thrombocytopenia, anaemia, hepatic dysfunction. FBC and LFTs should be monitored during treatment. ❗ ↓ anticoagulant effect of warfarin; interacts with allopurinol—dose of mercaptopurine should be ↓ if given concurrently.
Methotrexate Anti-metabolite (folic acid analogue) Given IV/ intra-thecally/ IM/PO	*Used for:* leukaemia, lymphoma, choriocarcinoma, head and neck cancers, breast cancer, sarcoma. *Toxicities:* myelosuppression; stomatitis; skin pigmentation; renal dysfunction (↑ Cr and haematuria). FBC and renal function should be monitored during treatment. ❗ Folinic acid (Leucovorin®) is incorporated into high-dose methotrexate regimens to ↓ severity of GI and bone marrow toxicity.
Mitomycin C Anti-tumour antibiotic Given IV/ intra-vesically	*Used for:* colorectal cancer, anal cancer in combination with radiotherapy, superficial bladder cancer. *Toxicities:* delayed myelosuppression—reaches maximum suppression ≈4wk after administration; thrombocytopenia; pulmonary fibrosis; haemolytic uraemic syndrome. FBC should be monitored during treatment.
Mitoxantrone Anti-tumour antibiotic Given IV	*Used for:* lymphoma, leukaemia, hormone-refractory prostate cancer. *Toxicities:* hair loss; myelosuppression; nausea/vomiting; cardiotoxicity; blue-green discolouration of sclera and/or urine.
Oxaliplatin DNA intercalating agent Given IV	*Used for:* colorectal cancer; upper GI malignancies. *Toxicities:* acute neurotoxicity (onset during or within hours of administration—paraesthesias of hands/feet, peri-oral area and/or choking sensation); chronic neurotoxicity (peripheral neuropathy—patients with diabetic neuropathy are more susceptible—resolves slowly on discontinuation of treatment); myelosuppression; nausea/vomiting; diarrhoea; pain at site of infusion; hypersensitivity reactions. *If pain develops in the infusion arm:* treat with simple analgesia. Inform oncology as slowing infusion rate during subsequent administrations prevents recurrence. ❗ Warn patients to avoid drinking ice-cold liquids around the time of administration and to wear gloves/scarfs in the cold due to cold-associated dysasthesia.

Table 4.7 (*Contd.*)

Agent	Indications and potential problems
Paclitaxel (*Taxol*®) Taxane (anti-microtubule agent) Given IV/PO	*Used for:* breast, ovarian, non-small cell lung, upper GI and head and neck cancers. *Toxicities:* hair loss; myelosuppression; peripheral neuropathy; fluid retention; stomatitis; nail changes (discolouration, separation from the nail bed); transient myalgia/arthralgia; hypersensitivity reactions (rash, flushing, low-back ache, anaphylactoid reactions with hypotension ± bronchospasm). Pre-medication with a 2d course of dexamethasone ↓ incidence of hypersensitivity reactions. *If myalgia/arthralgia develops:* give NSAID prn for pain relief—pain usually starts 2–3d after treatment and lasts for 2–4d. ⓘ Patients with diabetic neuropathy are more susceptible to drug-induced neuropathy.
Pemetrexed (*Alimta*®) Anti-metabolite (anti-folate drug) Given IV	*Used for:* non-small cell lung cancer; mesothelioma. *Toxicities:* myelosuppression; stomatitis; diarrhoea; drowsiness; rash. *If fever develops on treatment:* check FBC. If neutropenic (absolute neutrophil count <1.0×10⁹/l) refer for admission and antibiotics. ⓘ Vitamin supplementation with folic acid and B₁₂, ↓ toxicity.
Procarbazine Alkylating agent Given PO	*Used for:* lymphoma, brain tumour, myeloma. *Toxicities:* delayed myelosuppression (up to 4wk after treatment); thrombocytopenia; nausea/vomiting; rash. *If fever develops on treatment:* check FBC. If neutropenic (absolute neutrophil count <1.0×10⁹/L) refer for admission and antibiotics. ⓘ Late toxicities include infertility and ↑ risk of second malignancy.
Temozolomide Alkylating agent Given PO	*Used for:* malignant melanoma; brain tumour. *Toxicities:* myelosuppression; thrombocytopenia; nausea/vomiting; renal impairment; hyperglycaemia. FBC should be monitored during treatment.
Topotecan Topoisomerase I inhibitor Given IV	*Used for:* ovarian and small cell lung cancer. *Toxicities:* hair loss; myelosuppression; anaemia; nausea/vomiting; diarrhoea; headache. FBC should be monitored during treatment. *If fever develops on treatment:* check FBC. If neutropenic (absolute neutrophil count <1.0×10⁹/l) refer for admission and antibiotics.
Vinblastine Vinca alkaloid Given IV	*Used for:* lymphoma, leukaemia, germ cell tumours. *Toxicities:* myelosuppression; peripheral neuropathy; constipation; if extravasates causes blistering, ulceration ± tissue necrosis (*vesicant*). FBC should be monitored during treatment.

Table 4.7 (Contd.)

Agent	Indications and potential problems
Vincristine (Oncovin®) Vinca alkaloid Given IV	*Used for:* lymphoma, leukaemia, sarcoma. *Toxicities:* peripheral neuropathy; autonomic neuropathy; ataxia; if extravasates causes blistering, ulceration ± tissue necrosis (*vesicant*). 🔵 Patients with diabetic neuropathy are more susceptible to drug-induced neuropathy.
Vindesine Vinca alkaloid Given IV	*Used for:* leukaemia, malignant melanoma. *Toxicities:* myelosuppression; peripheral neuropathy; vesicant. FBC should be monitored during treatment. 🔵 Patients with diabetic neuropathy are more susceptible to drug-induced neuropathy.
Vinorelbine (Navelbine®) Vinca alkaloid Given IV/PO	*Used for:* Non-small cell lung cancer, breast cancer. *Toxicities:* Myelosuppression; constipation; fatigue; phlebitis of infused vein. FBC should be monitored during treatment. *If tenderness/discolouration of the infused vein:* supply topical/PO NSAID.

Figure 4.1 Action of cytotoxic chemotherapy on normal and cancer cell populations

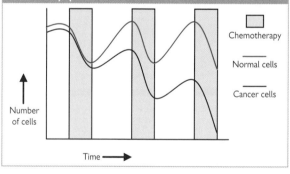

Advice for patients

Information about side effects of chemotherapy:

Chemocare 🖥 www.chemocare.com
Cancer Research UK ☎ 0808 800 4040 🖥 www.cancerhelp.org.uk
Macmillan Cancer Support ☎ 0808 808 0000
🖥 www.macmillan.org.uk

Table 4.8 Common biological agents: indications and side effects

Name and mode of action	Route	Indication	Common side effects
Bevacizumab (*Avastin®*) A monoclonal antibody that inhibits angiogenesis.	IV	Metastatic colorectal cancer and non-small cell lung cancer	Abdominal pain, headache, hypertension, diarrhoea, nausea, bleeding, thromboembolic events, and proteinuria
Bortezomib (*Velcade®*) A proteosome inhibitor, which is an enzyme system controlling cell function and growth.	IV	Multiple myeloma	Nausea, tiredness, constipation, decreased platelet blood count, fever, vomiting, peripheral neuropathy (may be painful)
Cetuximab (*Erbitux®*) A monoclonal antibody that blocks the epidermal growth factor receptor (EGFR).	IV	Metastatic colorectal cancer	Acneiform skin rash, nausea, diarrhoea, infusion-related hypersensitivity reactions, fever
Erlotinib (*Tarceva®*) A small molecule inhibitor of the EGFR tyrosine kinase.	PO	Non-small cell lung cancer	Skin rash, diarrhoea
Imatinib (*Glivec®*) 	PO	CML and gastro-intestinal tumours (GIST)	Fluid retention, skin rash, diarrhoea
Interferon-alfa An immunomodulatory agent.	IV/SC	Renal cancer, melanoma, carcinoid, myeloma	'Flu-like' symptoms (take 1g paracetamol before administration), headache, rash, fatigue, raised liver tests, depression
Interleukin-2 An immunomodulatory agent.	IV/SC	Renal cancer, melanoma	'Flu-like' symptoms, fluid retention, headache, rash, fatigue, raised liver tests
Rituximab (*MabThera®*) A monoclonal antibody that targets B-cell lymphocytes.	IV	Non-Hodgkin lymphoma	Infusion-related hypersensitivity reactions, reduced white blood cell counts
Trastuzumab (*Herceptin®*) A monoclonal antibody that targets the HER2 epidermal growth factor receptor.	IV	Early and advanced breast cancer	Infusion-related hypersensitivity reactions, nausea, cardiotoxicity, diarrhoea, headaches

Table 4.9 Hormone therapy			
Group	Agent	Indications	Common side effects
Anti-androgen	Bicalutamide Given PO	Locally advanced and metastatic prostate cancer	Hot flushes, gynae-comastia, impotence, hepatotoxicity
	Cyproterone acetate Given PO		
GNRH analogue	Buserelin Given SC or intra-nasally	Prostate and breast cancer	Hot flushes, gynae-comastia, impotence, nausea. Patients with implants may develop infection/bruising around the injection site
	Goserelin Implant		
	Leuprorelin Given IM		
Anti-oestrogens	Tamoxifen Given PO	Breast cancer in women of any age; primary prevention of breast cancer	Menopausal symptoms; thromboembolism; endometrial hyperplasia/carcinoma
	Fulvestrant Given IM	Metastatic post-menopausal breast cancer	Menopausal symptoms
	Anastrozole Given PO	Early and advanced postmenopausal breast cancer	Menopausal symptoms; arthralgia; ↑ fracture risk
	Exemestane Given PO		
	Letrozole Given PO		

Procedures

GPs are frequently asked by cancer patients what investigations or other procedures will entail for them.

Central venous access device (CVAD): Tube inserted into a central vein to enable easy administration of chemotherapy and/or fluids. They can also be used to take blood samples. There are two main types of CVAD:
- *Peripherally inserted central catheter (PICC)*—exit site at the elbow
- *Hickman catheter/line*—exit site at the clavicle/chest wall.

Insertion is done in secondary care. Once in place, CVADs require flushing and redressing 1×/wk. This can be done by the district nurse or a trained relative/friend of the patient. CVADs should be removed as soon as they are no longer required. This is also usually done in secondary care and should not be attempted by anyone without training to do so.

Potential problems:
- Infection—may present with systemic symptoms (fever, shivers etc.), as cellulitis, discharge on the dressing, or discharge from the line. Refer back urgently to the secondary care team looking after the patient
- Venous thrombosis—may present with superior vena cava obstruction (□ p.87), arm swelling, chest pain, or shortness of breath. If suspected refer urgently back to the secondary care team looking after the patient.

Gastrointestinal stent: Used to relieve GI obstruction in the oesophagus, duodenum, colon, or common bile duct. Positioned across the obstruction/compression in secondary care by a gastroenterologist or interventional radiologist.

Potential problems:
- Migration, blockage, or tumour overgrowth—may cause obstruction. Refer back to secondary care
- Pain—common for the first few days as stent dilates, but may be long-standing and require opioid analgesia.

Nephrostomy tube: Relieves ureteric obstruction by providing an external shunt for urine drainage from the renal pelvis. Insertion is performed in secondary care by an urologist/interventional radiologist.

Potential problems:
- Infection—check MSU and treat as appropriate if any symptoms/signs of infection e.g. fever, rigors, pain, offensive urine
- Pain—may be an indicator of blockage or infection—check renal function, MSU and treat infection. If no infection or passing very little or no urine, refer for check USS and/or urgent specialist opinion
- Tube has fallen out—refer back immediately to the secondary care team looking after the patient. If bleeding, advise the patient to apply pressure.

Ureteric stent: Used to relieve ureteric obstruction. It is positioned between the renal pelvis and bladder. Insertion is performed in secondary care by an urologist or interventional radiologist.

Common symptoms following stent insertion: Symptoms include the following:
- Frequency
- Urgency
- Haematuria
- Sensation of incomplete bladder emptying
- Stent colic.

Potential problems:
- Infection—check MSU and treat as appropriate if any symptoms/signs of infection e.g. frequency, urgency, dysuria, renal pain, fever
- Blockage—may present with pain and/or ↓ urine output. If suspected refer urgently to the secondary care team looking after the patient.

Advice for patients

Advice for patients with a:
Peripherally inserted central catheter (PICC):
- Wrap your arm in cling film to keep it dry while having a bath or shower
- Do not go swimming
- Ensure that your dressing stays on at all time
- Report any of the following symptoms to your oncology team
  - Redness or pain in your arm
  - Signs of infection such as feeling hot, shivery, or generally unwell or inflammation or discharge from the PICC
  - Fluid or blood under the dressing
  - Chest pain or shortness of breath
  - Swelling of your arm, neck or shoulder
  - If your PICC seems to be longer
  - If your PICC accidentally falls out—if you are bleeding apply pressure and call hospital immediately.

Hickman catheter: Report any of the following symptoms to your oncology team
- Redness or pain in your arm
- Signs of infection such as feeling hot, shivery, or generally unwell
- Inflammation or discharge from the Hickman catheter
- Fluid or blood under the dressing
- Chest pain or shortness of breath
- Swelling of your arm, neck, or shoulder.

Nephrostomy tube: Report any of the following symptoms to your doctor:
- Signs of infection such as feeling hot, shivery, or generally unwell
- Passing very little or no urine
- Increased pain
- Nephrostomy tube accidentally falls out—if you are bleeding apply pressure and call hospital immediately.

Ureteric stent: Report any of the following symptoms to your doctor:
- Signs of infection such as feeling hot, shivery, or generally unwell
- Passing very little or no urine
- Increased pain.

Further information:
Cancer Research UK ☎ 0808 800 4040 🖥 www.cancerhelp.org.uk
Macmillan Cancer Support ☎ 0808 808 0000
🖥 www.macmillan.org.uk

Paracentesis: This technique is used to reduce ascites for symptom control. Usually performed as an out-patient procedure—often after USS to localize best site and confirm that the procedure will be possible. Patients who have loculated ascities may have drain inserted under ultrasound guidance. If a patient has significant ascites, fluid may continue to drain after the tube has been removed. If the patient is clinically well then a stoma bag can be placed over the site to collect the continued drainage.

Potential problems:
- Infection—systemic symptoms/signs or local cellulitis
- Bleeding
- Damage to any intra-abdominal organ—usually bladder (results in haematuria) but can cause GI perforation.

In all cases, consult the secondary care team looking after the patient for advice on management.

Radiotherapy planning: Important to ensure that radiation is delivered to the tumour while sparing normal tissues. The planning session is usually done before commencement of treatment.
- The patient lies under a simulator. The simulator is similar to the treatment machine, but rather than giving treatment it takes X-rays to help plan the correct position for treatment. This procedure takes approximately 15–45min. On occasions, MRI or CT may be used instead
- Once the treatment area has been finalized, ink markings are usually made on the skin to pinpoint the exact place where the radiation is to be directed. Patients are advised how to look after these markings by the radiographers
- More commonly nowadays permanent, pinpoint, tattoo marks are also made on the skin.

Treatment to the pelvic area: To plan treatment to the pelvic area, contrast may be passed into the back passage or into the bladder, or a vaginal tampon may be used to show the exact position of the vagina.

Having a mask made for radiotherapy: As radiotherapy is planned very precisely, immobilisation is important to treat exactly the right area. A transparent perspex 'mould' or 'mask' may be made before treatment starts to prevent movement during treatment for head and neck areas. A plaster cast is made. Some patients find this claustrophobic. Then perspex is moulded to the cast to form the mask and holes are cut for the eyes, nose, and/or mouth. The mask is worn at the planning session and during treatment.

Positron emission tomography scan: Positron emission tomography (PET) measures metabolic activity in a tissue. Preparation required depends on the area being scanned. Before the scan, the blood sugar is checked and, if normal or minimally elevated, the patient is given a radioactive marker intravenously (usually fluorine 18 or FDG-18, a radioactive version of glucose). The patient then rests for about an hour to allow the radioactive tracer to spread through the body. The scan takes approximately 1h and detects areas of ↑ radioactive activity in areas where more of the radioactive marker is taken up.

🕕 The amount of radiation is very small—no more than that during a normal X-ray

Isotope bone scan: This scan is usually done in the medical physics or nuclear medicine department of the hospital. The scan involves one injection of a radioactive substance called a radionuclide which is given a few hours before the scan. Patients are advised to drink plenty of fluids after having the radionuclide injection.

During the scan, which takes about an hour, the patient lies still on an X-ray couch. The scan uses a 'gamma camera' that picks up radioactivity. The radionuclide collects in areas where there is a lot of activity in the bone—where bone is breaking down, or repairing itself—commonly called 'hot spots'.

It takes up to 24h for the radionuclide to get out of patients' systems and they are advised to drink plenty of fluids during this time.

⚠ PET scan or isotope bone scan patients should not have close contact with pregnant women, babies, and young children until the day after their scan.

Breastfeeding mothers are advised to express enough milk beforehand to get their baby through the first 6h after the scan. It is advisable that someone else feed the baby for 24h after the scan but it is safe to express more breast milk after 6h.

CHAPTER 4 **Principles of cancer treatment**

Complementary therapy

In the UK ≈90% of the population have tried complementary or alternative medicine (CAM) at some time. But, although CAM undoubtedly helps many individuals, its use remains controversial.

Reasons for caution

- *Lack of evidence of effectiveness:* There are many anecdotal reports and small scale observational studies of the positive effects of complementary therapies but large-scale, high-quality studies (which are rare) are mostly negative
- *Lack of regulation of practitioners:* Anyone can call themselves a therapist and practice. It is always important to find a reputable practitioner with accredited training who is a member of a recognized professional body. It is also important to ensure any practitioner carries professional indentity insurance
- *Lack of regulation of products:* Most complementary 'medicines' are sold as foods rather than medicines and do not hold a product license. No licensing authority has assessed efficacy, safety, or quality and interactions with conventional medicines are unknown. Complementary medicines can and frequently do cause adverse effects—just because they are natural does not mean they are safe.

Complementary therapy and cancer care: Complementary therapies are widely used by cancer patients—with and without their consultant's permission. There is very little evidence that any complementary therapies improve outcome.

Advantages of complementary medicine:
- Allows the patient to regain some control over their care
- May have soothing effects (e.g. aromatherapy massages, relaxation techniques) and thus improve quality of life for patients
- May alleviate symptoms (e.g. acupuncture for pain, tea tree oil dressings for offensive wounds)
- May alleviate side effects (e.g. acupuncture for chemotherapy-induced nausea).

Disadvantages of complementary medicine:
- Some practitioners insist patients stop conventional cancer treatment when they start complementary therapy
- Financial cost to the patient—private practitioners of complementary medicine may be expensive
- False hopes—patients may put their faith into unproven treatments and be disappointed when they fail
- Interaction with conventional treatment—complementary therapies (especially herbal medicines) may interact with conventional cancer treatments to cause additional toxicity and/or alter their effectiveness or with the patient's other medications.

Further information:

Bandolier ▣ www.jr2.ox.ac.uk/bandolier/booth/booths/altmed.html

Communication

Good communication with the patient, the family, and the other involved health and social-care workers is essential in cancer care (Box 4.1).

Stages of care:

- *Initial diagnosis:* Patients are shocked and may be in denial. Offer support to talk through the diagnosis, possible help available, and what will happen next
- *Staging and/or surgery:* Patients can struggle with uncertainty and therapeutic/prognostic information. Offer support but ensure that you do not give contradictory information as this can ↑ anxiety
- *Treatment:* Most support is provided by the oncology team. Keep up-to-date with treatment, likely side effects and follow-up plans
- *Relapse:* Knowledge that disease has progressed despite treatment is distressing for patients and families. Switching to palliative care can be difficult, often evoking feelings of abandonment. Provide additional support and continuity through the transition
- *Dying:* Honest, sensitive communication is essential. Be available and prepared to address spiritual concerns. Ensure there is co-ordination with out-of-hours services.

Answering questions about prognosis: This can be difficult. Contact the oncologist to find out their opinion if this is not clear from written communication. Emphasize that it is impossible to be accurate and talk in terms of day/weeks, weeks/months, and months/years. For example:

'When someone deteriorates from week to week, we are often talking in terms of weeks—although everyone is different'.

Useful questions include the following:
- What have the hospital doctors told you so far?
- What has prompted you to ask this question now?
- How do you see the situation?
- Are there any other specific issues, related to how long there is left on your mind that you would like to talk about?
- Are you the kind of person that likes to know everything?

Denial: Common coping mechanism which usually diminishes with time. Only if denial persists and interferes with care, is intervention required. However, may cause family distress and requires sensitive explanation.

Useful question to assess denial:
I know that you believe that you will beat this but is there ever a time, even for a moment, when you are not so sure?

Collusion: Relatives may request that patients are not told diagnosis/prognosis. Evidence suggests most patients do want to know to explain symptoms; make decisions about treatment; and organize their affairs.

Management:
- Acknowledge the family's anxiety
- Explain the reasons why patients wish to know their diagnosis
- Emphasize that patients usually guess from other clues anyway
- Stress the importance not to lie because of the breakdown of trust that this causes.

Box 4.1 Ten steps to breaking bad news

1 .*Preparation*
- Know all the facts before the meeting by reading all notes and correspondence
- Find out who the patient wants to be present
- Ensure comfort and privacy
- Minimize the risks of interruptions.

2. *What does the patient know?* Ask the patient for a brief narrative of events (e.g. how did it all start?).

3. *Give a warning shot:* 'I am afraid it looks rather serious'—then allow a pause for the patient to respond.

4. *Allow denial:* allow the patient to control the amount of information and proceed at their own pace.

5. *Explain (if requested) and check understanding:*
- Narrow the information gap step by step
- Use diagrams if the patient thinks they would be helpful
- Use appropriate language.

6. *Is more information wanted?*
- It can be very frightening to ask for more information and patients may not want to know any more!
- Test the waters by asking 'would you like me to explain a bit more?'

7. *Listen to concerns:* Ask, 'What are the things that bother you most at the moment?' This could be to do with physical or emotional health or relate to social or spiritual issues.

8. *Encourage ventilation of feelings*
- This conveys empathy and may be the key phase in terms of patient satisfaction with the interview
- Check that there is nothing else that they want to talk about.

9. *Summary and plan*
- Summarize concerns, plan treatment, and foster hope
- Check with the patient that they would have no objection for you to talk with the family either alone or with the patient.

10. *Offer availability*
- Most patients need further explanation (the details will not have been remembered) and support (adjustment takes weeks or months) and benefit greatly from a family meeting
- In addition, written material or a recording of the interview may be a useful adjunct to good communication.

Adapted from Kaye P. *Breaking Bad News.* Northampton: E.P.L. Publications, 1996.

GMS contract

Records 13	There is a system to alert the out-of-hours service or duty doctor to patients dying at home.	2 points

Chapter 5

Oncology emergencies

Bleeding

Large bleed: Make a decision whether the cause of the bleed is treatable or a terminal event.

Active treatment:
- Call for emergency ambulance support
- Lie flat and lift legs higher than body (e.g. feet on pillow)
- If haemoptysis, also protect airway and lie the patient on the bleeding side (if known) to protect the unaffected lung
- Gain IV access and give IV fluids if available. If possible take sample for FBC and cross-match on insertion.

No active treatment:
- Stay with the patient
- Give sedative medication (e.g. midazolam 10–40mg SC or IM, or diazepam 10–20mg PR)
- Support the carers
- Consider diamorphine 2–10mg SC if the patient is in pain.

Gastrointestinal bleeding: Bleeding due to cancer is usually due to a primary carcinoma of the stomach, oesophagus, or colon.

Presentation:
- Haematemesis—vomiting of blood—upper GI bleed
- Melaena—passage of black, offensive, tarry stool consisting of digested blood per rectum—usually upper GI bleed though may be due to haemoptysis if large amounts of blood are swallowed
- Passage of fresh red blood per rectal PR—usually lower GI bleed but very heavy upper GI bleeds can present with fresh red bleeding PR
- Faintness or dizziness especially on standing
- Patient feels cold or clammy
- Collapse ± cardiac arrest.

(!) Iron tablets may cause black stools.

Examination:
- Pulse—tachycardia
- BP—↓ and/or postural drop
- Jugular venous pressure —↓
- Vomitus

Management: If large bleed, manage as described earlier. If smaller, non-life threatening bleed, unless very frail, admit for further investigation and treatment. Palliative treatment options include laser treatment and arterial embolization—both can be performed on frail patients.

Haemoptysis: This is characterized by the expectoration of blood or blood-stained sputum. Bleeding due to cancer is most commonly from a primary carcinoma of the bronchus and a massive haemoptysis is usually from a squamous cell lung tumour lying centrally or causing cavitation. Small episodes of haemoptysis occasionally herald a catastrophic bleed. Although massive haemoptysis is rare, it is exceedingly distressing if it occurs.

(!) The patient is more likely to die from suffocation secondary to the bleed than from the bleed itself.

Management: If the patient is compromised by the bleeding (i.e. problems with airway, tachycardia, low BP, postural drop), treat as for large bleed (see opposite page). If not compromised by bleeding, reassure and monitor frequently. Consider:

- Checking FBC and clotting screen if on anti-coagulants or possible bleeding tendency. If low Hb, consider iron supplements/transfusion
- Treatment of infection that might exacerbate a bleed
- Minimizing bleeding tendency with tranexamic acide 1g tds po—stop if no effect after 1wk. If effective continue for 1wk after bleeding has stopped. Continue 500mg tds long term if bleeding recurs and responds to a further course of treatment. Weigh up benefits of stopping bleeding against ↑ risk of stroke or MI
- Referral to oncology for radiotherapy, chemotherapy, or palliative surgery (e.g. cautery).

Haematuria: This is a common symptom of bladder or prostate cancer. Large bleeds that cause circulatory compromise (low BP, tachycardia, postural drop) are rare—manage as described subsequently.

Management of non-life threatening bleeds:
- ↑ fluid intake to promote good urine output (helps avoid clot retention and clear UTI)
- Treat reversible causes e.g. UTI, bleeding tendency
- Stop drugs which might be causing/exacerbating bleeding
- If anaemic, consider iron supplements or transfusion
- Etamsylate 500mg qds may help by ↓ capillary bleeding in the bladder
- Bleeding from the prostate may respond to finasteride 5mg od
- Consider referral for palliative radiotherapy or surgery (cautery or iliac artery embolization).

✎ Use of tranexamic acid is controversial—it may cause formation of hard clots which then need to be irrigated cystoscopically.

Clot retention: This condition needs specialist management—admit. Specialist care involves evacuation of bladder clots. A non-distended bladder bleeds far less than a distended bladder.

Haemorrhagic cystitis: This is a side effect of chemotherapy with cyclophosphamide or ifosamide. Admit the patient.

Bleeding wounds: Prevent bleeding during dressing changes by:
- avoiding frequent dressing changes
- using non-adherent dressings or dressings which liquefy and can be washed off (e.g. Sorbsan®) and
- irrigating the wound with saline to remove dressings.

If there is surface bleeding—put pressure on the wound; if pressure is not working try:
- Kaltostat®
- adrenaline—1mg/ml or 1:1,000—on a gauze pad, or
- sucralfate liquid—place on a non-adherent dressing and apply firmly to the bleeding area.

Consider referral for radiotherapy or palliative surgery (e.g. cautery).

Venous obstruction

Deep vein thrombosis: Approximately 50% of patients with malignancy develop deep vein thrombosis (DVT)—most occur in the leg and 10% have symptoms. Other risk factors include the following:

- Age >40y
- COC/HRT use
- Smoking
- Recent trauma and/or surgery
- Obesity
- Immobility/recent long-distance travel
- PMH of thrombo-embolism or inherited clotting disorder
- Other medical conditions e.g. heart failure, nephrotic syndrome, Inflammatory bowel disease

Presentation: Unilateral leg pain, swelling, and/or tenderness ± mild fever, pitting oedema, warmth, and distended collateral superficial veins.

Differential diagnosis:

- Cellulitis
- Post-thrombotic syndrome
- Haematoma
- Acute arterial ischaemia
- Ruptured Baker cyst
- Lymphoedema
- Superficial thrombophlebitis
- Fracture
- Chronic venous insufficiency
- Hypoproteinaemia
- Venous obstruction

Investigation: Clinical diagnosis is unreliable.

- Only 50% of DVTs are symptomatic
- <50% with clinically suspected DVT have diagnosis confirmed on diagnostic imaging.

Relevance of active management of DVT in patients with advanced disease depends on the stage of the disease and symptoms. If active management is appropriate, refer for further assessment. Many hospitals have rapid access facilities for diagnosis bypassing conventional admission.

Specialist assessment: All patients with malignancy fall into a high-risk group and require USS. If USS is positive, diagnosis of DVT is confirmed.

- If USS is negative, USS is repeated after 1wk or the patient is assessed with venography, CT, or MRI.

Active management of patients with confirmed DVT:

- Initial anticoagulation is with low molecular weight heparin (LMWH) followed by oral anticoagulation (warfarin)—except if having chemotherapy when ongoing LMWH is preferred (↓ side effects/interactions)
- LMWH should be continued for at least 4d. and until INR is in the therapeutic range for ≥2d. Target INR is 2.5 (range 2–3).
- Anticoagulants ↓ risk of further thromboembolism and should be continued for 3–6mo after a single DVT.
- Graduated elastic compression stockings - ↓ risk post-thrombotic leg syndrome by 12–50%.

Pulmonary embolus: Venous thrombi—usually from a DVT—pass into the pulmonary circulation and block blood flow to the lungs.

⚠ Have a high level of suspicion. Patients may have minimal symptoms/signs apart from some pleuritic pain and dyspnoea.

Presentation:
- *Symptoms:* Acute dyspnoea, pleuritic chest pain, haemoptysis, syncope.
- Signs:
  - Hypotension
  - Tachycardia
  - Cyanosis
  - Tachypnoea
  - Pleural rub
  - ↑jugular venous pressure
- Look for a source of emboli—often DVT is not clinically obvious.

Differential diagnosis:
- Pneumonia and pleurisy
- MI/unstable angina
- Other causes of acute breathlessness—acute LVF, asthma, exacerbation of COPD, pneumothorax, shock (e.g. due to anaphylaxis), arrhythmia, hyperventilation
- Other causes of acute chest pain—aortic dissection, rib fracture, musculoskeletal chest pain, pericarditis, oesophageal spasm, shingles.

Management: Make a decision whether active management is appropriate. If a decision is made to actively treat, give oxygen, and admit as an acute medical emergency.

Specialist management: investigation to prove the diagnosis usually involves CT scanning nowadays but ventilation-perfusion (VQ) scan, MRI, and/or pulmonary angiography are occasionally used. If pulmonary embolus (PE) is proven, the patient is anti-coagulated. LMWH or warfarin should be continued for 3–6mo aiming to keep the INR ≈2.5 (range 2–3). Thrombolysis or surgery are rarely used.

Superior vena cava obstruction (SVCO): Results due to infiltration of the vessel wall, clot within the superior vena cava, or extrinsic pressure. 75% are due to 1° lung cancer. Lymphoma is the other major cause (15%). Occasionally SVCO is caused by thrombosis due to an indwelling central venous catheter.

Presentation: Usually develops insidiously over a number of weeks and presents with:
- Shortness of breath/stridor/hoarseness
- Headache worse on leaning forwards, stooping or lying flat ± visual disturbance ± dizziness/collapse
- Swelling of the face (particularly around the eyes), neck, hands, and arms, and/or injected cornea
- *Examination:* look for facial plethora, non-pulsatile distention of neck veins, and dilated collateral veins (small dilated veins over the anterior chest wall below the clavicles) in which blood courses downwards.

Management:
- Treat breathlessness (sit upright and give 60% oxygen)
- Treat pain/panic with opioids—5mg oral morphine solution 4 hourly ± benzodiazepine depending on the level of anxiety
- Start corticosteroid (dexamethasone 16mg/d)
- Refer urgently for oncology opinion. Palliative chemotherapy or radiotherapy has a response rate of 70% and ↓ symptoms in <2wk. Stenting ± thrombolysis is also an option. If secondary to an indwelling central venous catheter the patient is anti-coagulated and the catheter removed.

Neurological and orthopaedic emergencies

Raised intracranial pressure: Occurs with 1° or 2° brain tumours. Characterized by:

- Headache—worse on lying
- Vomiting
- Confusion
- Diplopia
- Convulsions
- Papilloedema.

Management:

- Unless a terminal event, refer patients urgently to neurosurgery for assessment. Options include insertion of a shunt or cranial radiotherapy
- If no further active treatment is appropriate start symptomatic treatment—raise the head of the bed, start dexamethasone 16mg/d (stop if no response in 1wk), and give analgesia.

Fitting: When the call for assistance is received, instruct the attendant:

- to stay with the fitting patient
- to move anything from the vicinity of the patient that might cause injury
- to turn the patient onto his/her side.

Immediate management on arrival:

- Ensure that the airway is clear
- Turn the patient into the recovery position (Figure 5.1)
- Prevent onlookers from restraining the fitting patient
- Do not give drugs for the first 10min—the fit is likely to stop spontaneously
- After 10min treat with diazepam 5–10mg IV or PR (5mg if 2–3y or elderly; 2.5mg if <2y).
- If the fit is not controlled treat as status epilepticus.

Status epilepticus: If >1 seizure without the patient regaining consciousness *or* fitting continues >20min:

- Give diazepam 5–10mg IV or PR (5mg if 2–3y or elderly; 2.5mg if <2y)
- Repeat every 15min until fits are controlled
- Check BM to exclude low blood sugar
- Unless in a very terminal state, arrange immediate admission even if fits are controlled.

Further management: If first fit, refer for further investigation.

Spinal cord compression: Affects 5% of cancer patients (10% of patients with spinal metastases)—70% in thoracic region. Presentation can be subtle. Maintain a *high* level of suspicion in all cancer patients who complain of back pain—especially those with known bony metastases or tumours likely to metastasize to bone. Most common in patients with lung, breast, or prostate cancer or multiple myeloma but increasingly seen with all tumours as survival improves.

Presentation:
- Often back pain ± tenderness, worse on lying down, coughing, sneezing, or straining, appears before neurology
- Neurological symptoms/signs can be non-specific—constipation, weak legs, urinary hesitancy
- Lesions above L1 (lower end of spinal cord) may produce UMN signs (e.g. ↑ tone and reflexes) and a sensory level
- Lesions below L1 may produce LMN signs (↓ tone and reflexes) and peri-anal numbness (cauda equina syndrome).

Management: Prompt treatment (<24–48h from first neurological symptoms) is needed if there is any hope of restoring function. Once paralysed, <5% walk again. Treat with oral dexamethasone 16mg/d. and refer urgently for assessment and surgery/radiotherapy unless in final stages of disease.

Bone fractures: Common in advanced cancer due to osteoporosis, trauma as a result of falls, or metastases. Have a low index of suspicion if a new bony pain develops.

⚠ In the elderly, fracture of a long bone can present as acute confusion.

Management:
- Give analgesia. Unless in a very terminal state, confirm the fracture on X-ray and refer to orthopaedics or radiotherapy urgently for consideration of fixation (long bones, wrist, neck of femur), and/or radiotherapy.

> ### Figure 5.1 The recovery position
>
>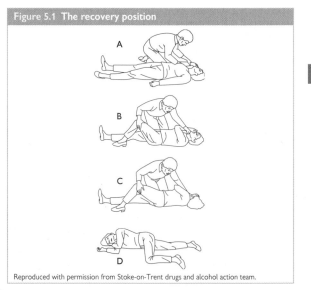
>
> Reproduced with permission from Stoke-on-Trent drugs and alcohol action team.

Other emergencies

Neutropaenic sepsis: Neutropaenic sepsis is defined as fever of ≥38.0°C for ≥2h when the neutrophil count is <1.0 × 10⁹/l. *Causes:*
- Chemotherapy (most common cause)
- Radiotherapy—if large volumes of bone marrow are irradiated e.g. pelvic radiotherapy
- Malignant infiltration of the bone marrow e.g. prostate/breast cancer

Risks of neutropenia: Bacterial and fungal infection. Risk of infection ↑ sharply as neutrophil counts fall below 1.0×10^9/l, with greatest risk at counts <0.1×10^9/l. Neutropenia for >5d is a further risk factor.

Presentation and primary care management: Symptoms/signs may be minimal—have a high index of suspicion. Neutropenic, septic patients can deteriorate rapidly and become hypotensive or moribund within hours. Early referral for hospital admission, investigation, and specialist management is critical.
- If a high-risk patient complains of chills, fever, rigors, sore throat, or generalized aches, check an urgent FBC
- Mouth ulcers and ↑ fatigue can be signs of neutropenia.

> ⚠ Development of fever in a patient with neutropenia is a medical emergency caused by infection until proven otherwise.

Specialist management: Initial management includes resuscitation if the patient is shocked and empirical broad-spectrum antibiotics. Antibiotic therapy may be modified later when causative organism and antibiotic sensitivities are identified. Second-line antibiotics or antifungal therapy are indicated if fever does not resolve in >48h. Granulocyte colony-stimulating factor may be administered to expedite neutrophil recovery during an acute episode of neutropenic sepsis or given prophylactically with subsequent cycles of chemotherapy.

Hypercalcaemia: Presence of ↑ corrected level of serum calcium (>2.6mmol/l). Occurs in 10% of patients with malignancy and particularly affects patients with:
- Myeloma (>30%) or breast cancer (40%)
- Other tumours which metastasize to bone—lung, kidney, thyroid, prostate, ovary, colon
- Squamous cell tumours.

GP notes

Checking Ca²⁺: Check calcium level on an *uncuffed* sample to avoid falsely high readings.

Correct for serum albumin—for every mmol/l less than 40, a correction of 0.02 mmol/l should be added to the serum calcium concentration measured. *For example:*

Calcium 2.40	Corrected Ca²⁺	= (40—24) × 0.02 + 2.4
Albumin 24		= 0.32 + 2.4 = 2.72

Presentation: It may be an incidental finding. Symptoms are non-specific:
- Tiredness, weakness, and lethargy
- Mild aches and pains
- Thirst, polydipsia, and polyuria
- ↓ appetite, nausea, and vomiting
- Abdominal pain
- Constipation
- Depression and/or confusion
- Stone formation or corneal calcification.

⚠ Always suspect hypercalcaemia if someone is iller than expected for no obvious reason. Untreated hypercalcaemia can be fatal.

Management: Depending on the general state of the patient, make a decision whether to treat the hypercalcaemia or not. If a decision is made not to treat, provide symptom control and don't check the serum calcium again. Active treatment depends on level of symptoms and Ca^{2+}. If the patient is asymptomatic with corrected calcium <3mmol/l, then monitor serum calcium levels and symptoms. If symptomatic and/or corrected calcium is ≥3mmol/l:
- Arrange treatment with IV fluids (as patient is profoundly dehydrated) and bisphosphonates via oncologist/palliative care team immediately
- Check serum calcium 7–10d post-treatment. 20% do not respond and there is no benefit from retreating them
- Effect of bisphosphonate lasts 20–30d. Consider maintenance with oral bisphosphonates started 1wk after the initial IV treatment or regular IV bisphosphonate. Many initially responsive to bisphosphonates become unresponsive with time.

Hyponatremia: Defined as serum sodium <130mmol/l. In cancer patients, usually due to syndrome of inappropriate anti-diuretic hormone (SIADH) due to ectopic antidiuretic hormone production by tumour cells, adrenal insufficiency, or drugs (e.g. cyclophosphamide, cisplatin).

Presentation: Often an incidental finding.
- Sodium <115 mmol/l—anorexia, lethargy, muscle cramps, weakness
- Sodium <110mmol/l—seizures, coma.

Management: Refer patients with symptoms urgently or as an emergency to oncology. Specialist treatment depends on cause.

Respiratory depression due to opioids:
- If respiratory rate ≥8/min and patient is easily rousable and not cyanosed—review if condition worsens. Consider reducing or omitting the next regular dose of opioid
- If respiratory rate <8/min and/or the patient is barely rousable/unconscious and/or cyanosed dilute a standard ampoule containing naloxone 400mcg to 10ml with sodium chloride 0.9%. Administer 0.5ml (20mcg) IV every 2min until respiratory status is satisfactory or until five doses have been given. If respiratory function still has not improved, question diagnosis.

🔔 Further boluses may be necessary once respiratory function improves as naloxone is shorter acting than morphine. Naloxone can cause severe exacerbation of pain previously treated with opioids that may be difficult to control. Contact the palliative care team, cancer centre, or hospice for specialist advice if this occurs.

Chapter 6

Specific cancers

Lung cancer

Second most common cancer (39,000 cases/y) and most common cause of cancer death in the UK. Incidence ↑ with age—85% are aged >65y and 1% <40y at presentation. ♂:♀≈2:1 but incidence is increasing in women (Figure 6.1).

Types:
- *Small cell lung cancer*—accounts for a quarter of all cases. Often disseminated by the time of diagnosis. Spreads to liver, bones, brain and adrenals.
- *Non-small cell lung cancer*—mainly adenocarcinoma or squamous cell carcinoma (SCC). Adenocarcinoma is not always related to smoking.

Screening: A 2003 Cochrane review concluded that current evidence does not support screening for lung cancer with chest radiography or sputum cytology. Frequent CXR screening might be harmful. Results of trials of screening with CT scanning are awaited from the US but preliminary results do not suggest any meaningful impact on cancer-related mortality.

Prevention:
- *Smoking cessation*—90% of lung cancer patients are smokers or ex-smokers. The younger a person is when s/he starts smoking the greater the risk of developing lung cancer. Risk also ↑ with amount smoked (duration of smoking and daily number of cigarettes smoked)
- *Diet*—↑ consumption of fruit, carrots and green vegetables may ↓ incidence but there is no evidence that vitamin supplements are beneficial and they might be harmful[C].

Presentation: More than 90% have symptoms at the time of diagnosis. Common presenting features:

- Cough (56%)
- Chest/shoulder pain (37%)
- Haemoptysis (7%)
- Dyspnoea
- Hoarseness
- Weight ↓
- Finger clubbing
- General malaise
- Distant metastases
- Incidental finding on CXR.

Pancoast syndrome: Apical lung cancer + ipsilateral Horner syndrome (miosis, ptosis, and loss of hemifacial sweating).

Cause: invasion of the cervical sympathetic plexus.

Other features: shoulder and arm pain (brachial plexus invasion C8-T2) ± hoarse voice/bovine cough (unilateral recurrent laryngeal nerve palsy and vocal cord paralysis).

Paraneoplastic syndromes: Affect 10%–20% of patients with lung cancer—particularly small cell—Table 6.1. Have a high index of suspicion and refer for specialist management if suspected.

Management: Once the diagnosis has been confirmed, liaise with the chest physician, specialist lung cancer team, primary health-care team, and specialist palliative care services (e.g. Macmillan Nurses). Active treatment options depend on type and extent of tumour and include surgery, radiotherapy, and/or chemotherapy (Table 6.2 and 6.3, 📖 p.101). Follow-up regularly. 80% die in <1y.

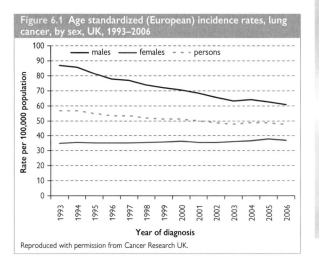

Figure 6.1 Age standardized (European) incidence rates, lung cancer, by sex, UK, 1993–2006

Reproduced with permission from Cancer Research UK.

Table 6.1 Paraneoplastic syndromes associated with lung cancer
Syndrome
Endocrine—usually due to ectopic hormone production
• Hypercalcaemia
• Cushing syndrome (due to ectopic ACTH production)
• Hyponatremia (syndrome of inappropriate ADH)
• Hyperthyroidism.
Skin, bone, and soft tissue
• Dermatomyositis   • Finger clubbing
• Acanthosis nigricans   • Hypertrophic pulmonary osteoarthropathy.
Neuromuscular—due to immune response to tumour
• Peripheral neuropathy   • Eaton Lambert (myaesthenic) syndrome
• Cortical cerebellar degeneration
• Retinopathy   • Polymyositis
• Autonomic neuropathy.
Other
• Nephrotic syndrome
• Hypercoagulability (thrombophlebitis migricans).

Palliative radiotherapy: Radiotherapy is a key component of symptomatic treatment for:
- Haemoptysis
- Chest pain
- Breathlessness due to bronchial occlusion
- Pain from bone metastasis
- Symptoms from brain metastases.

Radiotherapy may be combined with palliative chemotherapy, particularly for patients with non-small cell lung cancer.

Mesothelioma: This can follow even limited exposure to asbestos. There is often a 20–40y time lag between exposure and appearance of disease. Presents with increasing shortness of breath ± pleuritic pain. Examination and CXR reveal unilateral (rarely bilateral) effusion. Combination chemotherapy only helps a small minority and radiotherapy may be useful in some for palliation. Median survival is 2y from diagnosis.

❶ Patients with mesothelioma are eligible for Industrial Injuries Benefit in the UK (📖 p.203). Deaths of all patients with mesothelioma must be notified to the coroner.

Further information:

NICE 🖥 www.nice.org.uk
- Referral guidelines for suspected cancer—quick reference guide (2005)
- Lung cancer: diagnosis and management (2005)

Advice for patients
Information and support for patients: **Lung cancer resources directory** 🖥 www.cancerindex.org **The Roy Castle Lung Cancer Foundation** 🖥 www.roycastle.org **Macmillan Cancer Support** ☎ 0808 808 0000 🖥 www.macmillan.org.uk **British Lung foundation** ☎ 08458 50 50 20 🖥 www.lunguk.org

GMS contract			
Cancer 1	The practice can produce a register of all cancer patients defined as a 'register' of patients with a diagnosis of cancer excluding non-melanotic skin cancers from 1.4.2003.	5 points	
Cancer 3	% of patients with cancer, diagnosed within the last 18mo who have a patient review recorded as occurring within 6mo of the practice receiving confirmation of the diagnosis.	Up to 6 points	40%–90%
Education 7	The practice has undertaken a minimum of 12 significant event reviews in the past 3y which could include (if these have occurred) new cancer diagnoses.	Total of 4 points for 12 significant event reviews	

Table 6.2 Staging and prognosis of non-small cell lung cancer

Staging

Tumour		Lymph nodes involved		Metastases	
T1	≤3cm diameter	N0	No	M0	No spread beyond the affected lobe
T2	Tumour >3cm diameter *or* Involves main bronchus *or* Involves visceral pleura	N1	Involvement of local LNs	M1	Spread outside the affected lobe
T3	Lung collapse due to tumour or Invasion of chest wall, mediastinal pleura, diaphragm, *or* pericardium	N2	Involvement of ipsilateral hilar or mediastinal LNs		
T4	Mediastinal invasion or Malignant pleural effusion	N3	Involvement of contralateral or supraclavicular LNs		

Prognosis

Stage		TNM equivalent	Treatment	5y survival
1	A	T1, N0, M0	Surgical resection where possible.	80%
	B	T2, N0, M0		60%
2		T1/2, N1, M0 or T3, N0, M0	Radical radiotherapy ± chemotherapy is an alternative if the tumour is inoperable or the patient unfit.	40%–50%
3		Any T or N, M0	Surgery	25%–30%
			Radiotherapy + chemotherapy	7%–17%
			Radiotherapy alone	5%–10%
4		Any T or N, M1	Supportive care, chemotherapy and/or palliative radiotherapy.	2%*

*15%–35% 1y survival with chemotherapy; 10% 1y survival without chemotherapy.

Table 6.3 Staging and prognosis of small cell lung cancer

Stage	Definition	Prognosis
Limited disease (33%)	Local disease with no spread beyond local LNs	With chemotherapy: 35%–40% 2y survival.
Extensive disease (67%)	Distant spread	Without chemotherapy—survival in weeks. With chemotherapy—average survival 10–12mo

Breast cancer

Breast cancer is now the most common cancer in the UK—>100 women are diagnosed with the disease every day (1:9 women in their lifetime). Men can also get breast cancer but it is rare (1% of female cases).

Risk factors:

Geography: This is more common in the developed world—migrants assume the risk of the host country within two generations.

Personal characteristics:
- *Age*—↑ with age—~80% of breast cancers occur in women >50y
- *Socioeconomic status*—higher incidence in more affluent social classes
- *Physical characteristics*—taller women have ↑ risk; women with denser breasts have 2–6× ↑ risk.

Lifestyle factors:
- *Obesity*—↑ risk after menopause
- *Physical activity*—30% ↓ risk if taking regular physical activity
- *High-fat diet*—probably associated with ↑ risk
- *Alcohol*—↑ risk by 7%/unit consumed/d.

Reproductive history:
- *Early menarche or late menopause* -↑ risk
- *Pregnancy*—↑ parity → ↓ risk (32% ↓ risk in women having three births compared to women having no births); late age when first child is born ↑ risk
- *Breastfeeding*—↓ relative risk by 4.3% for each year of breastfeeding.
- *Combined oral contraceptive*—slight ↑ risk (relative risk 1.24 for current users)—excess risk disappears within 10y. of stopping
- *HRT*—risk ↑ by 6 cases/1,000 after 5y combined HRT use and 19 cases/1,000 after 10y use. Risk for combined oestrogen and progesterone preparations is >oestrogen only preparations. HRT also ↓ sensitivity of mammography.

Other past medical history:
- *Past history of breast disease*—ductal or lobular carcinoma *in situ*, florid hyperplasia, and papilloma with fibrovascular core all ↑ risk
- *Ionizing radiation*—exposure ↑ risk.

Family history: Referral algorithm—Figure 2.4, 📖 p.27
- *One first-degree relative with breast cancer (mother or sister)*—↑ risk × 2—but 95% of women with breast cancer have no family history
- *Several family members with early onset breast cancer*—refer for genetic screening—*BRCA1* and *BRCA2* genes account for 2%–5% all breast cancers.

Prevention:
Consider referral to secondary/tertiary care if family history of breast cancer.
- Lifestyle measures—↓ alcohol intake; ↓ weight; avoid exogenous sex hormones (e.g. HRT); breast feed
- Chemoprophylaxis—tamoxifen ↓ risk of breast cancer by 40% in high-risk women but use is limited by side effects (thromboembolism and endometrial carcinoma)—other drug trials are in progress with agents with less side effects
- Prophylactic surgery—↓ risk by 90% in very high risk women.

Patient experiences of diagnosis of breast cancer:

'The fact is I was so shocked because I wasn't expecting it whatso-
ever that I didn't do anything. I just sat deadly still and I didn't know
what to do. It was awful because no one was there and then they
went out the room and they went into the office and they left me on
my own in that little room and that's when I burst into tears. That's
when, that's when the reality hit me.'

'And people's reactions to it were, (cancer) sort of: 'Ughhh!', you
know. They don't like, I mean a lot of people just don't like mention-
ing the word. . . And, sometimes I felt some people avoided me
because they didn't know what to say. So that was, that was hard to
bear really I think. I mean some people were great but some people,
and I mean it wasn't that people didn't want to help, they just didn't
know what to say. And so they just avoided it. And avoided me,
which was difficult.'

Patient experience of worries over body image:

'You know how most men have a favourite part of the anatomy, my
husband's happens to be the breast. So I did think that that would be
difficult for him and me, if I ever talk to him about it now all he'll say
is that he would rather have me with one breast or no breast than
not have me at all. But that's what he says to me, I don't think that is
necessarily what he thinks. . . But it's, you still feel rejected in a way
because you just feel that it can't be the same any more no matter
how much he says that it doesn't matter, because it must matter, it
must make a difference.'

Breast cancer information and support:
Patient experience database—☐ www.healthtalkonline.org
Breakthrough breast cancer: ☐ www.breakthrough.org.uk
Breast Cancer Care ☎ 0808 800 6000
☐ www.breastcancercare.org.uk
Breast Cancer Campaign ☐ www.bcc-uk.org
Against Breast Cancer ☐ www.aabc.org.uk
CancerHelp UK ☎ 0808 800 4040 ☐ www.cancerhelp.org.uk
Macmillan Cancer Support ☎ 0808 800 0000
☐ www.macmillan.org.uk

Lympoedema information and support:
Lymphoedema support network ☎ 020 7351 4480
☐ www.lymphoedema.org/lsn
UKLymph.com On line support network ☐ www.uklymph.com
Skin Care Campaign ☐ www.skincarecampaign.org
CancerHelp UK ☎ 0808 800 4040 ☐ www.cancerhelp.org.uk

Patient experiences are reproduced with permission from the DIPEx patients experience
database ☐ www.healthtalkonline.org.

Breast cancer screening: 📖 p.24.

Presentation: Often found at breast screening (📖 p.24). Clinical presentations include:
- Breast lump (90%)
- Breast pain (21% present with painful lump; pain alone <1%)
- Nipple skin change (10%). Any red, scaly lesion, or eczema around the nipple suggests *Paget disease of the breast*—intraepidermal, intraductal cancer
- Family history (6%)
- Skin contour change (5%)
- Nipple discharge (3%)
- Rarely presents with distant metastases e.g. bone pain
- In the elderly, may present with extensive local lesions.

Management:
- Refer for urgent assessment (<2wk) to a breast surgeon
- Specialist investigation includes mammography, USS ± fine needle aspiration, or core biopsy
- If diagnosis is confirmed further investigations include tumour markers, and/or CT/MRI, liver USS and/or bone scan to evaluate spread.

Treatment: Is determined by the stage (Table 6.4) and type of tumour. It includes surgery (lumpectomy ± axillary clearance, mastectomy), endocrine therapy, radiotherapy, and/or chemotherapy.

Adjuvant endocrine therapy: Oestrogen has an important role in the progression of breast cancer. Oestrogen and progesterone receptors determine the response to endocrine therapy.
- *Tamoxifen*—↑ survival of patients with oestrogen receptor +ve tumours (60% tumours) of any age but rarely causes endometrial cancer—warn patients to report any untoward vaginal bleeding. Continue tamoxifen for ≥5y—take advice from a specialist before stopping
- *Anastrozole* (Arimidex®)—blocks peripheral synthesis of oestrogens. Superior efficacy when compared to tamoxifen for post-menopausal women with hormone sensitive early breast cancer and first choice drug for post-menopausal women with advanced breast cancer. Continue for ≥5y—take advice from a specialist before stopping
- *Trastuzumab* (Herceptin®)—monoclonal antibody directed against HER2, a receptor found in 1:5 breast cancers. Affects division and growth of breast cancer cells. Treatment option for women with early HER2 +ve cancer at high risk of recurrence and women with advanced HER2 +ve breast cancer. Administered IV every 3wk for 1y.

🚨 Optimum treatment regimes for breast cancer change regularly and there are regional variations. Many women will be asked to participate in clinical trials to answer important questions on improving efficacy and decreasing side effects.

Psychological impact of breast cancer: Depression, anxiety, marital, and sexual problems are common. Be sensitive. Discuss possibilities of reconstructive surgery or breast prostheses as appropriate. Refer to the specialist breast care nurse for support and advice.

Table 6.4 Classification of breast cancer stage

Stage	TNM Equivalent	Features
In situ	Tis N0 M0	Non-invasive.
Stage I	T1 N0 M0	≤2cm diameter. No LNs affected. No spread beyond breast.
Stage II	T0–2 N1 M0 or T2/3 N0 M0	2–5cm diameter and/or LNs in axilla involved. No evidence of spread beyond axilla.
Stage III	T0–2 N2 M0 or T3 N1/2 M0 or T4 any N M0 or Any T N3 M0 or	>5cm diameter. LNs in axilla involved. No evidence of spread beyond the axilla.
Stage IV	Any T/N M1	Any sized tumour. LNs in axilla may be affected. Distant metastases.

Virtually all breast cancers are adenocarcinoma (85% ductal; 15% lobular)

GP notes

Sentinel lymph node (LN) biopsy: Prognosis and decisions surrounding adjuvant treatment are based on knowledge of the axillary node status. The only way to assess axillary LN involvement is to remove nodes surgically and look at them under the microscope. Axillary node clearance can result in lymphoedema and reduced arm function. Sentinel node biopsy is the removal of the key or sentinel LN in patients undergoing surgery for early breast cancer to accurately predict the state of nodal disease in the remaining axillary LNs. Radical axillary surgery to clear the axillary nodes can then be reserved for the 20%–40% with a +ve sentinel LN biopsy.

Further information:

NICE 🖥 www.nice.org.uk
- Improving outcomes in breast cancer (2002)
- Classification and care of women at high risk of familial breast cancer in primary, secondary and tertiary care (2006)
- Breast cancer: diagnosis and treatment (2009)

Clinical Evidence 🖥 www.clinicalevidence.com
- Stebbing et al. Breast cancer (metastatic) (2006)
- Rodger et al. Breast cancer (non-metastatic) (2005)

Cancer Research UK Breast cancer survival statistics
🖥 www.cancerresearchuk.org/cancerstats
Cochrane Badger et al. Physical therapies for reducing and controlling lymphoedema of the limb (2004)
Adjuvant online—decision making tool for professionals. assessing risks and benefits of additional therapy after surgery
🖥 www.adjuvantonline.com

Prognosis:

- 72% of women diagnosed now will live 10y; 64% live ≥20y.
- Recurrence is most likely <2y after treatment—late recurrences do occur but the longer since diagnosis, the less the chance of recurrence
- Prognosis for a given individual depends on age (patients aged 50–69y have best prognosis), stage of disease (Figure 6.2), grade of tumour, HER2, and oestrogen receptor status (both HER2 +ve and oestrogen receptor -ve tumours have poorer prognosis). Women who live in affluent areas have better survival rates than women in deprived areas.

Lymphoedema: Results from obstruction of lymphatic drainage resulting in oedema with high-protein content. In patients with breast cancer it usually affects one arm but may also affect both arms and/or head and neck.

Risk factors: ↑ with age; obesity; lack of physical exercise.

Causes: Axillary involvement or treatment of breast cancer (axillary surgery, post-operative infection, or radiotherapy).

Presentation:
- Swollen limb ± pitting—Figure 6.3
- Impaired limb mobility and function
- Discomfort/pain related to tissue swelling and/or shoulder strain
- Neuralgia pain—especially when axillary nodes are involved
- Psychological distress.

Management: Untreated lymphoedema becomes increasingly resistant to treatment due to chronic inflammation and subcutaneous fibrosis.

- *Avoid injury:* In at risk patients (e.g. patients who have had breast cancer with axillary clearance) or those with lymphoedema, injury to the limb may precipitate or worsen lymphoedema. Avoid sunburn and cuts (e.g. wear gloves for gardening). Do not take blood from the limb or use it for IV access, vaccination, or BP measurement
- *Skin hygiene:* Keep the skin in good condition with moisturizers e.g. aqueous cream; treat fungal infections with topical agents e.g. clotrimazole cream
- *Cellulitis* is a common complication and causes rapid ↑ in swelling. Treat with oral antibiotics (e.g. penicillin V 500mg qds). If ≥2 episodes of cellulitis consider prophylactic antibiotics e.g. phenoxymethylpenicillin V 250mg bd
- *External support:* Intensive support can be provided with special compression bandages—refer to specialist physiotherapy or the palliative care team. Maintenance therapy with a lymphoedema sleeve is helpful—contact the palliative care team or breast care specialist nurse for information
- *Exercise:* Advise gentle daily exercise of the affected limb, gradually increasing range of movement. ❶ Patients should wear their compression bandages or lymphoedema sleeve whilst doing their exercises.
- *Massage:* Very gentle finger tip massage in the line of drainage of the lymphatics can help—refer to specialist physiotherapist for advice
- *Diuretics:* If condition develops/deteriorates after corticosteroid or NSAID use, or if there is a venous component, consider trial of diuretics e.g. furosemide 20mg od. Otherwise diuretics are of no benefit.

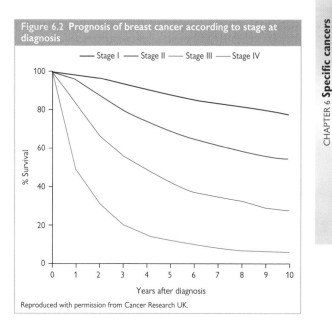

Figure 6.2 Prognosis of breast cancer according to stage at diagnosis

Reproduced with permission from Cancer Research UK.

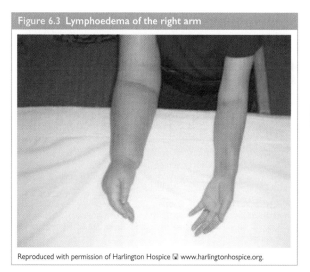

Figure 6.3 Lymphoedema of the right arm

Reproduced with permission of Harlington Hospice 🖳 www.harlingtonhospice.org.

Ovarian cancer

Ovarian tumours: May be solid or cystic. In women of reproductive age, >80% are benign. The remainder are borderline or malignant. In postmenopausal women, the proportion of malignant ovarian tumours rises to ~50%. Classified according to tissue of origin:

- Tumours of surface epithelium—60%—Table 6.5
- Germ cell tumours—15%–25%
- Gonadal stromal tumours—5%–10%
- Metastatic (from breast, stomach, colon or genital tract)—5%–10%.

Presentation: Tends to present late and with advanced disease. Early tumours are often asymptomatic and may be an incidental finding on pelvic examination done for another reason (e.g. when doing a cervical smear) or on USS. Symptoms include:

- Non-specific—weight ↓/cachexia, constipation, early satiety, fatigue
- Abdominal pain—rapidly expansion of tumour, rupture, torsion, infection, or bleeding.
- Abdominal distension/bloating—tumour or ascites
- Pressure effects e.g. urinary retention/urinary frequency, prolapse
- Menstrual disturbance
- Endocrine effects—due to hormone production by tumour.

ⓘ In the UK, ~80% of patients with ovarian cancer have had symptoms for <4wk before seeing their GP.

Initial management: If suspected, refer for urgent USS.

- If USS is suggestive of ovarian cancer, check CA125 and refer urgently to gynaecology (to be seen in <2wk)
- If a child (pre-menarchal)—refer any cyst >2cm diameter
- If pre-menopausal—refer any cysts with multi-locular or solid elements, cysts >8cm diameter, or cysts <8cm that fail to regress in <6wk
- If post-menopausal—refer any cyst/ovarian mass.

Screening: Ovarian cancer fulfils some of the criteria necessary for the introduction of population screening—it is an important health problem, and early detection is associated with improved outcomes. Although both USS and serum tumour markers (e.g. CA125) can detect a significant proportion of ovarian cancers pre-clinically, there is no evidence that early detection through screening ↓ mortality. To clarify this issue, two large scale trials of screening are underway in the UK:

UK Familial Ovarian Cancer Screening Study—5,000 women aged >35y with a significant family history of ovarian cancer. Screening involves annual CA125 measurement and USS.

UK Collaborative Trial of Ovarian Cancer Screening—200,000 post-menopausal women. Screening tests used are annual CA125 and/or transvaginal USS. Encouraging early results were published in 2009, due to be completed in 2010.

Table 6.5 Tumours of surface epithelium

Type of tumour	Subtype	10y survival
Serous Peak age 30–40y; 20%–50% ovarian tumours; 30% bilateral	Benign serous cystadenoma—60% of serous tumours; 25% of all benign ovarian tumours.	100%
	Borderline serous cystadenoma—10% of serous tumours.	90%–95%
	Malignant serous cystadenocarcinoma—25%–50% of serous tumours; bilateral in 40%–60%; 40%–50% all malignant ovarian tumours; 85% have spread outside the ovaries at the time of diagnosis; >50% are >15cm diameter at diagnosis.	15%
Mucinous Can be very large; often multi-locular; often contain viscid mucin—if burst can cause pseudomyxoma peritonei (mucin secreting cells are spread throughout the peritoneum).	Benign mucinous cystadenoma—peak incidence aged 30–50y; 80% of mucinous tumours; bilateral in 5%–10%; 20%–25% of all benign ovarian tumours.	100%
	Borderline mucinous cystadenoma—10% mucinous tumours; bilateral in 10%.	90%–95%
	Malignant mucinous cystadenocarcinoma—peak age 40–70y; 10% of mucinous tumours; bilateral in 15%–30%; 5%–10% of all 1° ovarian cancers; average diameter at diagnosis ≈16cm.	34%

Endometrioid
Peak age 50–60y; 30%–50% bilateral; benign tumours are rare; malignant tumours account for 20%–25% of all malignant ovarian neoplasms; 30% co-exist with endometrial cancer; 10% co-exist with endometriosis.

Clear cell (mesonephroid)
5% bilateral; 5%–10% of all malignant ovarian neoplasms; 25% co-exist with endometriosis; associated with hypercalcaemia.

Brenner (transitional cell)
Rare—2%–3% of all ovarian tumours; >90% are benign. If malignant, have poor prognosis; <5% are bilateral; associated with mucinous cystadenoma and cystic teratoma in 1:10 cases.

Undifferentiated carcinoma
<10% epithelial neoplasms; no histological features that characterize it.

Further information:
NICE Referral guidelines for suspected cancer (2005)
🖳 www.nice.org.uk
SIGN Epithelian ovarian cancer (2007) 🖳 www.sign.ac.uk
Cancer Research UK Ovarian cancer statistics
🖳 www.cancerresearchuk.org/cancerstats
Clayton, Monga & Baker *Gynaecology by Ten Teachers* Hodder Arnold (2006) ISBN: 0340816627

Epithelial ovarian cancer (EOC): Approximately 90% of ovarian cancers. ~7,000 cases are diagnosed each year in the UK (2.5% of all cancers) and ovarian cancer accounts for 6% of ♀ deaths. Median age at diagnosis is 66y. Incidence is rising.

Risk factors:
- *Age*—peak age 50–70y; 85% ovarian cancers occur in ♀>50y.
- *Family history*—Mutations in *BRCA1*, *BRCA2*, and hereditary non-polyposis colorectal cancer (*HNPCC*) genes are associated with ↑ risk of ovarian cancer, although only 10% of ovarian cancers occur in women carrying these mutations. Women who have inherited a gene mutation that puts them at high risk of ovarian cancer may consider having prophylactic surgery (bilateral oophorectomy) which reduces but does not abolish their risk. Regular screening (with USS and CA125) for the early signs of ovarian cancer is currently only available as part of a research study in the UK
- *Nulliparity*—odds ratio 2.42 compared to women with ≥4 children
- *Infertility*—odds ratio for women trying to conceive for >5y = 2.67 compared to women trying to conceive for <1y—this is probably *not* an effect of infertility drugs
- *Obesity* may ↑ risk.

Protective factors:
- *Pregnancy*—the more pregnancies, the lower the risk
- *COC*—↓ risk by ~60%. Protective effect is maintained >20y after the COC has been discontinued
- *Breastfeeding*—may ↓ risk by 20%
- *Tubal ligation*—↓ risk by 30%–70%
- *Hysterectomy*—may ↓ risk.

Treatment: Specialist management is with laparotomy ± adjuvant treatment with chemotherapy dependant on stage of disease. Chemotherapy and rarely radiotherapy may be used for palliation. Staging and prognosis—Table 6.6

Gonadal stromal tumours: Derived from the mesenchymal stroma of the gonad. Usually present early with symptoms of hormone production. All are rare. Treatment is surgical.

Types:
- *Granulosa cell tumours:* Most common. May be non-functional or secrete oestrogens. Associated with endometrial cancer in adults due to unopposed oestrogen secretion. Prognosis is good
- *Thecomas:* >65% occur in post-menopausal women. Usually secrete oestrogen (rarely virilizing). Often, tumours have both granulosa and thecal elements—granulosa-theca cell tumours
- *Fibromas:* Benign tumours consisting of fibrous tissue. Do not secrete anything. May occur in association with pleural effusion (*Meig syndrome*) ± ascites. Mechanism is not understood
- *Sertoli cell and Leydig cell tumours or Leydig cell (lipid cell tumours)*—very rare. Usually androgenic and/or virilizing.

Table 6.6 Stage and prognosis of ovarian cancer

Stage		Sub-stage		5y survival
I	Tumour confined to the ovaries (20% new diagnoses)	A	Tumour limited to one ovary.	73%
		B	Tumour limited to both ovaries.	
		C	IA or IB with tumour on external surface of the ovary, ruptured capsule or malignant cells in ascites or peritoneal washings.	
II	Tumour involving one or both ovaries with pelvic extension	A	Extension and/or implants in uterus and/or fallopian tubes.	34%
		B	Extension to other pelvic organs.	
		C	IIA or IIB with malignant cells in ascites or peritoneal washings.	
III	Tumour involving one or both ovaries with microscopically confirmed perito-neal metastases outside the pelvis and/or regional lymph node metastases	A	Microscopic peritoneal metasta-ses outside the pelvis.	27%
		B	Peritoneal metastases ≤2cm diameter outside the pelvis.	
		C	Peritoneal metastases >2cm diameter outside the pelvis and/or pelvic, para-aortic or inguinal lymph node metastases.	
IV	Distant metastases (40% new diagnoses)			16%

GMS contract			
Cancer 1	The practice can produce a register of all cancer patients defined as a 'register' of patients with a diagnosis of cancer excluding non-melanotic skin cancers from 1.4.2003.	5 points	
Cancer 3	% of patients with cancer, diagnosed within the last 18mo who have a patient review recorded as occurring within 6mo of the practice receiving confirmation of the diagnosis.	Up to 6 points	40%–90%
Education 7	The practice has undertaken a minimum of 12 significant event reviews in the past 3y which could include new cancer diagnoses	4 points	for 12 reviews

Germ cell tumours: These arise from the germ cell elements of the ovary. Types are as follows:

- *Mature teratoma (or ovarian dermoid cyst):* Benign; 25% of all ovarian tumours; bilateral in 20%. Peak age at diagnosis is 20–30y. Frequently an incidental finding. May contain skin, hair, cartilage, bone, or other structures. Rarely secrete thyroxine if thyroid tissue is present within the cyst and can cause hyperthyroidism. Usually removed surgically. Rarely malignant change can occur in older women

- *Immature teratoma:* Malignant tumour. Rare—<1% of ovarian teratomas but 20% of malignant germ cell tumours. Presents in the first two decades of life. Usually unilateral. ↑ serum αFP (used as tumour marker). Treated with surgery and chemotherapy. 5y survival 60%–90%

- *Dysgerminoma:* 30%–40% malignant germ cell tumours (1%–3% of ovarian cancers). Peak incidence aged >10y and <30y. Unilateral in 85%–90%. Highly sensitive to radio- and chemotherapy. Placental alkaline phosphatase (PLAP) is used as a tumour marker. 5y survival rate ~95%

- *Endodermal sinus tumour (yolk sac tumour):* Overall 20% malignant germ cell tumours. Unilateral in 95%. Tends to be fast growing and presents with an acute abdomen. ↑ serum αFP (used as a tumour marker). 5y survival 60%–70%

- *Rare tumours:* Embryonal carcinoma, choriocarcinoma, and gonadoblastoma. Associated with ↑ αFP and/or ↑ β-human chorionic gonodotropin (HCG) (both are used as tumour markers). All are treated with surgery and chemotherapy. Overall 5y survival is ~60%.

⊙ Mixed germ cell tumours account for ~10% of malignant germ cell tumours—usually contain dysgerminoma and endodermal sinus tumour.

Advice for patients

Experiences of women with ovarian cancer:

Symptoms:

'Ovarian cancer is called the 'silent killer' for a reason because, you know, I think women always have pains and because I was reaching menopausal age I really kind of thought these pains were related to my ovaries drying up or, you know, your body going through the change because you expect that. . . you tend to incorporate those pains and not necessarily think that they're linked so something that's, you know, worrying.'

'And I really hadn't felt ill, I'd lost a lot of weight before that, but I'd had a year of [stress] . . . and, so I'd put all my weight loss down to that. And that was the only real indication that I had that anything was wrong with me.'

Diagnosis:

'In beginning I told them they must be dreaming, it cannot happen to me, because in my family there's nobody who has ever had it. Even up to this day I believe it's a dream, and to me it's a dream, it's a bad bad dream.'

'Well, the consultant showed me the scan of this little cauliflower thing and he told me what it was and I felt quite calm, actually. Just sat there, I suppose because it really didn't sink in and he told me what would happen with me; I'd go in, have the operation, have both ovaries out and some lymph glands. And I drove home quite calm and it wasn't until I came in the street door that it suddenly hit me, and I just burst into tears.'

Adjusting after treatment:

'I think I left hospital and I really was aware that despite being told that everything looks like it's going to be fine, they can't say a hundred percent but it looked really good and the prognosis was great. I felt absolutely terrified and I knew that there was a huge kind of conflict between what I was being told and what I felt.'

Ovarian cancer information and support:

Ovacome ☎ 0845 371 0554 ▢ www.ovacome.org.uk
DIPEx Patient experience database ▢ www.healthtalkonline.org.uk
Cancer Research UK (CancerHelp) ☎ 0808 800 4040
▢ www.cancerhelp.org.uk
Macmillan Cancer Support ☎ 0808 808 8000
▢ www.macmillan.org.uk

Patient experiences are reproduced with permission from ▢ www.healthtalkonline.org.uk

Other gynaecological cancers

Cervical intraepithelial neoplasia: Invasive carcinoma of the cervix is preceded by pre-malignant lesions. The vast majority of these changes are detected in women <45y. with peak incidence in the 25–29y age group. Cervical intraepithelial neoplasia (CIN) is a histological diagnosis resulting from biopsy—usually following an abnormal smear.

Classification:
- CIN 1   Nuclear atypia confined to basal one third of the epithelium (mild/moderate dysplasia)
- CIN 2   Nuclear atypia in basal two thirds of the epithelium
- CIN 3   Nuclear abnormalities through the full thickness of the epithelium (severe dysplasia/carcinoma *in situ*).

Natural history: Unclear. CIN 1 may revert to normality. Any stage can progress to cervical cancer—although more likely with CIN 3.

Treatment: Depends on stage and ranges from local ablation (diathermy, laser diathermy, cold coagulation) through large loop excision of the transformation zone (LLETZ), and cone biopsy to hysterectomy. Excisional techniques are preferred as tissue is preserved for histology.

Cervical cancer: In the UK, each year 2,800 women are diagnosed with cervical cancer (2% of all female cancers). There are two peaks of incidence—women in their late 30s and women in their 70s/80s (Figure 6.4). 80% have squamous cell cancer—the remainder adenocarcinoma. Incidence is dropping probably due to the cervical cancer screening programme and changes in sexual practices.

Risk factors:
- Social class
- Smoking
- Early age of 1st intercourse
- Early age of 1st pregnancy
- Multiple sexual partners
- HPV infection (types 16, 18, 31, 33)
- History of dyskaryosis
- Method of contraception (↓ with barrier methods; ↑ if >5y COC use)
- Immunosuppression, HIV.

Presentation:
- Routine cervical screening—📖 p.20
- Post-coital, inter-menstrual, or post-menopausal bleeding
- Offensive vaginal discharge
- Cervical ulceration/mass or cervix which bleeds easily.

Management: Refer urgently to gynaecology. Treatment is with surgery ± radiotherapy depending on the stage of the disease:
- *Stage 1:* microinvasive cancer (A)/cancer confined in the cervix (B)—5y survival 70%–95%
- *Stage 2:* invasion into the upper third of the vagina (A) or parametria (B) but not to the pelvic side wall. 5y survival 60%–90%
- *Stage 3:* Extension to the lower third of the vagina (A) or pelvic side wall (B). 5y survival 30%–50%
- *Stage 4:* tumour involving bladder/rectum (A) or extra-pelvic spread (B). 5y survival 20%–30%.

>65% of women present with stage 1 cancer so overall 5y survival is 64%. <6% of cervical cancer deaths occur in women <35y mainly because they tend to be diagnosed at an early stage.

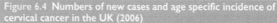

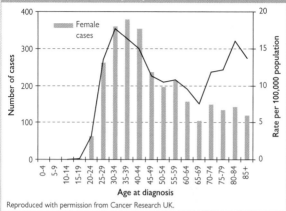

Figure 6.4 Numbers of new cases and age specific incidence of cervical cancer in the UK (2006)

Reproduced with permission from Cancer Research UK.

Advice for patients

Patient experiences of discovering their cervical cancer:

'I hadn't had a cervical smear for quite a while because like a lot of women I don't particularly like having them and it had just sort of lapsed. So I thought well I'd better go and have one done. Which I did at my local GP and it came back with some abnormalities and, surface abnormalities.

So they asked me to go to hospital to have a colposcopy which I'd never had before and that was really awful as I'm sure a lot of women would know. Sort of the full examination lights, cameras, action and all the rest of it. And I found that quite traumatic. But I went to see the consultant at the hospital afterwards for the results and I went on my own. And the consultant said that they'd found, not just abnormalities on the surface but actual cancer cells deeper down in the neck of the womb.'

'I was angry and I felt it wasn't fair. Had I never ever been for a smear in my life I would've have thought well tough you've brought this on yourself and maybe if you'd been, you wouldn't be in this mess now. But when I'd been very diligent and it was just 18 months ago that it was totally clear, to suddenly have a tumour. I felt it was grossly unfair, I didn't want it.'

Cervical cancer information and support:

Patient experience database ▢ www.healthtalkonline.org
Cancer Research UK (CancerHelp) ☎ 0808 800 4040
▢ www.cancerhelp.org.uk
Macmillan Cancer Support ☎ 0808 808 0000
▢ www.macmillan.org.uk

Patient experiences are reproduced with permission from ▢ www.dipex.org.uk

Endometrial carcinoma: Approximately 7,000 women each year are diagnosed with endometrial cancer in the UK (4% of all female cancers). It is predominantly a disease of post-menopausal women with 93% of cases diagnosed in women >50y (peak age 61y).

Risk factors:
- Age
- Obesity
- Nulliparity
- Late menopause
- Diabetes mellitus
- Drugs—unopposed oestrogen, tamoxifen
- Granulosa cell ovarian tumour
- Family history -breast, ovary, or colon cancer
- Previous pelvic irradiation.

Risk is ↓ with current or past use of the COC pill and/or progestogens.

Presentation: Postmenopausal bleeding (PMB) (>90%)—any woman presenting with a PMB has endometrial carcinoma until proven otherwise. Pre-menopausally tends to occur in overweight women and presents with continual bleeding. Rarely may be detected on routine cervical smear.

Management: Refer any PMB to gynaecology for further investigation. Assessment comprises transvaginal USS to look at endometrial thickness ± endometrial sampling with pipelle or hysteroscopy.

Treatment: TAH and BSO ± radiotherapy, progestogen therapy, and/or chemotherapy depending on stage and differentiation of the tumour. Staging and prognosis—Table 6.7.

Vaginal cancer: Rare. Occurs in the sixth or seventh decade. 90% are squamous cell cancer—the rest are clear cell (associated with in utero exposure to stilboestrol), 2° tumours or sarcomas. Present with postmenopausal bleeding. Most are treated with radiotherapy though surgery is an option in the early stages. Refer all women with post-menopausal bleeding for prompt gynaecological assessment.

Vulval intraepithelial neoplasia: Vulval intraepithelial neoplasia (VIN) may be associated with other genital tract neoplasia (e.g. CIN 📖 p.110). Presents with abnormal looking skin of the vulva (usually pinkish white and altered texture) ± white patches ± itch. Diagnosis is histological following skin biopsy:
- VIN 1   Epidermis is thickened. Atypia is confined to the basal third of the epithelium
- VIN 2   Nuclear atypia in the lower half of the epithelium
- VIN 3   Carcinoma *in situ*—nuclear atypia through the full thickness of the epithelium.

Management: Refer all patients with abnormal looking vulval skin (without candidal infection or other obvious cause) to gynaecology for skin biopsy and treatment. Treatment depends on site, histology, and extent—includes observation with regular biopsies, surgery, cryocautery, laser vaporization, or topical chemotherapy.

Vulval carcinoma: Rare. Mainly affects women in their eighth decade. Most are SCC; others—melanoma, basal cell carcinoma (BCC), Bartholins gland carcinoma, and adenocarcinoma. The majority occur on the labia and spread to local LNs. Present early with chronic pruritus vulvae (>66%), vulval lump, or ulcer. Refer for confirmation of diagnosis. Treatment is surgical.—5y survival rate ≈95%.

Table 6.7 Stage and prognosis of endometrial cancer

Stage		Sub-stage	
I	Cancer confined to the corpus uteri	A	Tumour limited to endometrium.
		B	Invasion to <50% of the myometrium.
		C	Invasion to >50% of the myometrium.
II	Cancer involves the corpus and the cervix but has not extended outside the uterus	A	Endocervical glandular involvement only.
		B	Cervical stromal invasion.
III	Cancer extends outside the uterus but is confined to the pelvis	A	Tumour invades the serosa and/or adnexa and/or positive peritoneal cytology.
		B	Vaginal metastases.
		C	Metastases to pelvic and/or para-aortic LNs.
IV	Cancer involves the bladder or bowel mucosa or has meta-stasized to distant sites	A	Tumour invasion of bladder and/or bowel mucosa.
		B	Distant metastases, including intra-abdominal and/or inguinal LNs.

Grade

G1: ≤5% of a non-squamous or non-morular growth pattern
G2: 6%–50% of a non-squamous or non-morular growth pattern
G3: >50% of a non-squamous or non-morular solid growth pattern

Survival: depends on age of the patient, stage and grade—overall 10y survival is 75%.
Stage I tumours—5y survival 85% (grade 1 stage IC—81%; grade 3 stage IC—42%).
Stage IV tumours—5y survival 25%.

GMS contract

Cancer 1	The practice can produce a register of all cancer patients (excluding non-melanotic skin cancers) from 1.4.2003.	5 points	
Cancer 3	% of cancer patients, diagnosed ≤18mo ago who have a patient review recorded as occurring <6mo after the practice received confirmation of diagnosis.	Up to 6 points	40%–90%
Education 7	The practice has undertaken a minimum of 12 significant event reviews in the past 3y which could include new cancer diagnoses.	4 points	for 12 reviews

Advice for patients

Information for patients:
Hysterectomy Association 🖳 www.hysterectomy-association.org.uk
Cancer research UK (Cancer Help) 🖳 www.cancerhelp.org.uk

Further information:
SIGN Management of cervical cancer (2008) 🖳 www.sign.ac.uk
RCOG Management of vulval cancer (2006) 🖳 www.rcog.org.uk

Prostate cancer

Prostate cancer is the second most common cancer worldwide. In the UK, it is the most common cancer affecting men and 10,000 men die from the disease every year. 1:10 men have clinical prostate cancer in their lifetimes and incidence is rising.

Risk factors:
- *Age:* Uncommon <50y; 85% of men with prostate cancer are diagnosed aged >65y.
- *Genetic:* ↑ incidence if first-degree relative affected
- *Racial:* Incidence varies according to location in the world and ethnic group. Highest rates are in men of black ethnic group in the US—lowest in Chinese men
- *Dietary:* Links are proposed between prostate cancer and low intake of fruit (particularly tomatoes) and high intake of fat, meat and Ca^{2+}.

Symptoms and signs:

Early cancer: Symptomless. Often detected after an incidental finding of ↑ PSA. A hard nodule is sometimes felt in prostate on rectal examination.

Local disease:
- Prostatism
- Urinary retention
- Haematuria
- Lower extremity oedema
- On rectal examination, the prostate is hard, non-tender, and sulci lose definition.

Metastatic disease:
- Malaise
- Weight loss
- Bone pain
- Pathological fractures
- Spinal cord compression
- Ureteric obstruction may cause renal failure
- Signs depend on site of metastases.

Investigation: A digital rectal examination and a PSA test (after counselling—📖 p.31) are recommended for patients with any of the following unexplained symptoms:
- Inflammatory or obstructive lower urinary tract symptoms
- Erectile dysfunction
- Haematuria
- Lower back pain
- Bone pain
- Weight loss, especially in the elderly.

🚫 Exclude UTI before PSA testing, and postpone rectal examination until after the PSA test is done. Interpretation of PSA results—📖 p.33.

Urgent referral: To be seen in <2wk by an urologist.
- Rectal examination—hard, irregular prostate typical of prostate cancer. PSA result should accompany the referral
- Rectal examination—normal prostate, but rising/raised age-specific PSA ± lower urinary tract symptoms*
- Symptoms and high PSA levels
- For asymptomatic men with borderline, age-specific PSA results, repeat the PSA test after 1–3mo If PSA level is rising, refer urgently.

*Consider discussion with specialist and patient (and/or carer) before referral if very elderly or compromised by other co-morbidities.

GMS contract				
Cancer 1	The practice can produce a register of all cancer patients defined as a 'register' of patients with a diagnosis of cancer excluding non-melanotic skin cancers from 1.4.2003.	5 points		
Cancer 3	% of patients with cancer, diagnosed within the last 18mo who have a patient review recorded as occurring within 6mo. of the practice receiving confirmation of the diagnosis.	Up to 6 points	40%–90%
Education 7	The practice has undertaken a minimum of 12 significant event reviews in the past 3y which could include (if these have occurred) new cancer diagnoses.	Total of 4 points for 12 significant event reviews		

Advice for patients

Information about PSA testing and prostate cancer:

National screening 🖳 www.cancerscreening.nhs.uk

Macmillan Cancer Support ☎ 0808 808 0000
🖳 www.macmillan.org.uk

Prostate cancer charity ☎ 0800 074 8383
🖳 www.prostate-cancer.org.uk

Prostate cancer support association ☎ 0845 601 0766
🖳 www.prostatecancersupport.co.uk

Further information for GPs:

NICE 🖳 www.nice.org.uk
- Improving outcomes in urological cancers (2002)
- Referral guidelines for suspected cancer (2005)

Cancer research UK 🖳 www.cancerresearchuk.org

Symptomless local disease: Treatment is controversial. There are two views:

| Benefits of treatment are outweighed by risks | or | Aggressive treatment before spread is the only way to ensure cure. |

The picture is further complicated as >50% of men >50y who die from other causes are found post-mortem to have prostate cancer—prostate cancer kills only a small minority of men who have it. The personal and economic cost of treating men whose cancer would never have caused them any problems must be considered.

Options:

- *Watchful waiting:* Monitor with PSA/rectal examination. ↑ in PSA or size of nodule triggers active treatment. At 10y follow-up <10% with moderately well-differentiated cancer will have died from their cancer. Progression rates are higher in patients with poorly differentiated cancer. Some men find the uncertainty of waiting difficult to cope with
- *Radical prostatectomy:* Has potential for cure, but in the age group most affected by prostate cancer, mortality is 1.4%. Other common complications: impotence (50%), incontinence (25%)
- *Radiotherapy:* May not be effective—persistent cancer is found in 30% on biopsy. Brachytherapy (localized radioactive treatment using implanted seeds or wires) has proven efficacy in early prostate cancer
- *Hormone treatment:* No convincing evidence that this gives survival benefit in early disease other than in use with radical radiotherapy
- *Others:* Other minimally invasive treatments e.g. cryotherapy and microwave therapy are as yet unproven.

Symptomatic disease: 30% 5y survival. Hormone manipulation is the mainstay of treatment and gives 80% ↓ in bone pain, PSA, or both and a lower incidence of serious complications (e.g. spinal cord compression) if treatment starts at the time of diagnosis. *Options:*

Luteinizing hormone releasing hormone (LHRH) analogues: e.g. goserelin—SC injection every 4–12 wk (depending on preparation used). Testosterone levels ↓ to levels of castrated men in <2mo. *Side effects:* impotence, hot flushes, gynaecomastia, local bruising and infection around injection site. When starting LHRH analogues, LH level initially ↑ which can cause ↑ tumour activity or 'flare'. Counteracted by prescription of anti-androgens (e.g. flutamide) for a few days before administration of the first dose of LHRH and concurrently for 3wk. Response in most patients lasts for 12–18mo.

LHRH antagonists: e.g. degarelix. This has advantages including much more rapid reduction in testosterone levels, reduction in testosterone-induced flare, and maintenance of castrate levels of testosterone.

Anti-androgens: e.g. cyproterone acetate, flutamide, bicalutamide. Anti-androgens do not suppress androgen production completely. Used to prevent side effects due to testosterone flare during initiation of LHRH analogues, as monotherapy in those who find LHRH analogues unsuitable (flutamide 250mg tds—monitor liver function if used long term), and in combination with LHRH analogues to maximize androgen blockade.

Surgical castration: ↓ testosterone secretion permanently without the need for medication. It has cheap and fewer side effects than other options, but rarely used now in the UK.

Bony metastases: In addition to hormone therapy, local radiotherapy and corticosteroids are used for bone pain. Radioactive strontium ↓ the number of new sites of bone pain developed. Mean survival is <5y.

Hormone resistant disease: No agreed treatment. There is some evidence that prednisolone 5mg daily or diethylstilboestrol 3mg daily is helpful. Many new agents are undergoing clinical trials in this setting and early results are encouraging with improvements in symptom-control, quality of life, and possibly in survival.

Prognosis: Table 6.8.

Table 6.8 Features affecting prognosis of prostate cancer

Stage

Tumour		Lymph nodes involved?		Metastases?	
T1	Inpalpable.	N0	No	M0	No spread outside the pelvis.
T2	Tumour completely within the prostate gland.	N1	1 +ve LN <2cm diameter	M1	Spread outside the pelvis.
T3	Tumour has breached the capsule of the prostate.	N2	>1 +ve LN or 1 LN of 2–5cm diameter		
T4	Spread within the pelvis e.g., to bladder or bowel.	N3	Any +ve LN > 5cm diameter		

Gleason score: Histological grade. Cells are graded 1–5 the less differentiated they are. The two areas of the biopsy with the highest grade cells are added together. Low-grade tumours likely to grow slowly have low scores (2–4); high-grade tumours have high scores (7–10).

Age: Older patients with low-grade tumours are likely to die from something other than their prostate cancer.

PSA:
- PSA > 40—high chance of nodal or metastatic spread
- PSA > 100—metastatic spread is very likely.

Prognosis: 5y survival rates for tumour stage:
- 1 or 2: tumour confined within the prostate—65%–98%
- 3: tumour has breached the capsule of the prostate—60%
- 4: spread to LNs, within the pelvis or elsewhere—20%–30%.

Other urological cancers

Bladder cancer: Incidence: 1:5,000; $\male:\female \approx$ 3:1. Transitional cell carcinoma (TCC) is most common in the UK—squamous cell carcinoma (SCC) is most common worldwide.

Risk factors:
- Smoking (half of the male cases are attributable to smoking)
- Aromatic amine exposure (textile or rubber industries)
- Schistosomiasis (SCC)
- Chronic UTI.
- Stasis of urine

Presentation: Haematuria—painless or painful. *Less commonly:*
- Recurrent UTI
- Pelvic pain
- Frequency
- Bladder outflow obstruction.
- Loin pain

Investigation: MSU—excludes UTI and detects sterile pyuria and/or microscopic haematuria.

Management: Refer urgently to urology. Most urology departments have one-stop haematuria clinics offering rapid out-patient assessment of haematuria. Treatment depends on stage at diagnosis—Table 6.9.

Hypernephroma: Clear cell adenocarcinoma of renal tubular epithelium. *Typical age:* 50y. $\male:\female \approx$ 2:1. Spread can be local or haematogenous (bone, liver, lung—causes cannon ball metastases seen on CXR).

Presentation:
- Haematuria
- Left varicocoele
- Loin pain
- Anaemia
- Abdominal mass
- Occasional night sweats.

Investigations:
- *Urine:* Red blood cells
- *Blood:* ↑ packed cell volume (2%), anaemia, hypercalcaemia
- *Radiology:* USS, CXR.

Management: Refer to urology urgently. Treatment includes nephrectomy ± immunotherapy with interferon and interleukin-2. 30%–50% 5y survival. Recently, sunitinib (an orally administered anti-angiogenic drug) has been licensed in the advanced disease setting and is associated with significant improvement in survival and quality of life.

Carcinoma of the penis: SCC (95%) or malignant melanoma. Usually in elderly men. Rare in the UK. Refer urgently patients with symptoms or signs of penile cancer. These include:
- Progressive ulceration in the glans, prepuce or skin of the penile shaft
- Mass in the glans, prepuce, or skin of the penile shaft

🛈 Lumps within the corpora cavernosa can indicate Peyronie disease which does not require urgent referral

Treatment involves surgery or radiotherapy. The majority are cured.

Carcinoma of the scrotal skin: SCC or melanoma. Uncommon <50y. Presents with a painless lump or ulcer of the scrotal skin ± enlarged inguinal LNs. If suspected, refer urgently for specialist management to urology or dermatology. Specialist treatment—📖 p.150.

Table 6.9 Stage of bladder cancer, treatment, and prognosis

Stage	Description and treatment	Prognosis
T1 (80%)	Disease confined to mucosa/submucosa. Treated with TURBT ± single intravesical chemotherapy treatment. Follow-up is with regular cystoscopy.	Very good prognosis—most die from other causes.
T2	Invasion into connective tissue surrounding the bladder. Treatment is with TURBT ± radiotherapy. Follow-up as for T1.	60% survive 5y
T3	Invasion through the muscle into the fat layer. Radical cystectomy and/or radiotherapy.	40%–50% 5y survival.
T4	Spread beyond the bladder. TURBT for local symptoms. Palliative radiotherapy ± chemotherapy. Palliative care.	20%–30% 5y survival—less if para-aortic nodes are involved.

GMS contract

Cancer 1	The practice can produce a register of all cancer patients defined as a 'register' of patients with a diagnosis of cancer excluding non-melanotic skin cancers from 1.4.2003.	5 points	
Cancer 3	% of patients with cancer, diagnosed within the last 18mo who have a patient review recorded as occurring within 6mo of the practice receiving confirmation of the diagnosis.	Up to 6 points	40%–90%
Education 7	The practice has undertaken a minimum of 12 significant event reviews in the past 3y which could include (if these have occurred) new cancer diagnoses.	Total of 4 points for 12 significant event reviews	

Advice for patients

Information and support for patients:
Macmillan Cancer Support ☎ 0808 808 0000
🖥 www.macmillan.org.uk
Cancer Research UK ☎ 0808 800 4040 🖥 www.cancerhelp.org.uk

Further information:

NICE 🖥 www.nice.org.uk
● Improving outcomes in urological cancers (2002)
● Referral guidelines for suspected cancer (2005)
● Sunitinib for the first-line treatment of advanced and/or metastatic renal cell carcinoma (2009)

Cancer Research UK 🖥 www.cancerresearchuk.org

Testicular cancer: Most common malignancy in men age 20–34y devastating disease as sufferers tend to be young and fit and don't expect to be ill. Screening is not effective. Education to ensure men check their testes for lumps regularly and present early is preferable.

Risk factors:
- Undescended testes—bilateral undescended testis → 10× ↑ risk
- Past history testicular cancer—4% risk of second cancer.

Presentation:
- Painless lump in testis
- Occasional testicular pain or secondary hydrocoele
- May present with metastases—back pain/dyspnoea.

Types of testicular cancer: See Table 6.10.

Management: Testicular lumps are tumours until proven otherwise. Refer for urgent urological opinion. USS can help diagnosis but *don't* delay referral. Definitive diagnosis is only made at biopsy.

Specialist treatment depends on tumour type and extent. Sperm banking is routinely offered before therapy in case of ↓ fertility due to treatment. Cytotoxic chemotherapy has revolutionized the care of men with these tumours, with huge improvements seen in survival.

ⓘ Children conceived of men treated for testicular cancer are not at ↑ risk of congenital abnormality.

Table 6.10	Types and features of testicular cancer	
	Seminoma (60%)	**Teratoma**
Typical age	30–40y	<30y
Tumour markers	None	β-hCG α-FP LDH—correlates with volume of metastatic disease
Nature of tumour	Solid	Solid/cystic components. 40% occur within seminomas. Mixed tumours are treated like teratomas.
Speed of growth	Slow growing	Fast growing—can double in size in days.
Stage of presentation	90% stage 1 (tumour confined to testis)	60% stage 1 (tumour confined to testis).
Treatment	Treated with inguinal orchidectomy and radiotherapy. Relapses are treated with chemotherapy. More advanced disease is treated with radio- or chemotherapy.	Treatment of stage 1 disease is with inguinal orchidectomy and surveillance of tumour markers. 25% relapse in <18mo. Treatment of relapses and metastatic disease is with chemotherapy.
Survival	98% 5y survival for stage 1 disease. Overall >85% 5y survival.	Prognosis depends on stage and degree of differentiation.

Advice for patients

Testicular self-examination:

Who should examine their testicles? All boys aged above 14 years, and men should examine their testicles each month. In this way they will become familiar with the normal feel of their testicles, and be able to spot any abnormalities that arise.

When should I examine my testicles? Testicular self-examination is best performed after a warm bath or shower as heat relaxes the scrotum making it easier to spot anything unusual.

How should I examine my testicles?
1. Stand in front of a mirror. Check for any swelling on the scrotal skin
2. Examine each testicle with both hands. Place the index and middle fingers under the testicle with the thumbs placed on top. Roll the testicle gently between the thumbs and fingers—you should not feel any pain. Don't be alarmed if one testicle seems slightly larger than the other, that's normal
3. Find the epididymis, the soft, tube-like structure behind the testicle that collects and carries sperm.

What abnormalities am I looking for? Testicular cancer usually appears as a painless lump on the testicle. Lumps on the epididymis are not cancerous. Other things to watch out for are:
• Any enlargement of a testicle
• A significant loss of size in one of the testicles
• A feeling of heaviness in the scrotum
• A dull ache in the lower abdomen or in the groin
• A sudden collection of fluid in the scrotum
• Pain or discomfort in a testicle or in the scrotum
• Enlargement or tenderness of the breasts.

If you are not sure what is normal, compare one testicle with the other. It is very unusual to get testicular cancer in both testes at once.

What should I do if I find a lump or if I am worried about any other symptom? Make an appointment to see your GP as soon as possible. Only 4 in every 100 lumps found turn out to be cancer, so the abnormality may not be cancer. But if it is, then early treatment is often curative. When in doubt, get it checked out—if only for peace of mind!

Further information:
Cancer Research UK ☎ 0808 800 4040 ▣ www.cancerhelp.org.uk

GP notes

Undescended testis: Observed in 2%–3% of male neonates but most descend during the first year. Refer those that don't for surgical descent and fixation to avoid later infertility and ↑ risk of malignancy.

Upper gastrointestinal cancer

Carcinoma of the oesophagus: Common cancer accounting for 7,000 deaths/y in the UK. Most common in patients >60y. Overall ♂:♀ ≈ 2:1 (Figure 6.5). Usually presents late when prognosis is poor. There are two types:
- SCC (50%)—predominant form in upper two thirds of the oesophagus
- Adenocarcinoma (50%)—predominant in lower third of the oesophagus. Incidence is increasing. ♂:♀ ≈ 5:1.

Common risk factors:

SCC—account for 89% of cases
- Smoking*
- Alcohol
- Low fruit/vegetable intake

Adenocarcinoma—account for ~9% of cases
- Smoking*
- Obesity
- Low fruit/vegetable intake
- Gastro-oesophageal reflux—particularly Barrett's oesophagus (risk ↑ >30×—the longer the affected segment, the higher the risk).

* Risk ↓ to that of a non-smoker 10y after giving up.

Other risk factors:
- Previous mediastinal radiotherapy (↑ ×2 for patients treated for breast cancer; ↑ × 20 for patients treated for Hodgkin's lymphoma)
- Plummer–Vinson (or Patterson–Kelly) syndrome—oesophageal web and iron deficiency anaemia
- Tylosis—rare, inherited disorder with hyperkeratosis of the palms—40% develop oesophageal cancer.

Presentation:
- Usually presents with a short history of rapidly progressive dysphagia affecting solids initially then solids and liquids ± weight loss ± regurgitation of food and fluids (may be blood stained). Retrosternal pain is a late feature. Other symptoms include hoarseness and/or cough (due to aspiration or fistula formation)
- Examination may be normal. Look for evidence of recent weight loss, hepatomegaly and cervical lymphadenopathy.

Management: Refer for urgent endoscopy if the diagnosis is suspected. Rapid access dysphagia clinics run in many areas. Classified as operable type, locally advanced, or metastatic at presentation. Specialist management involves potentially curative radical resection or radical chemoradiotherapy (treatments of choice with similar efficacy but only 1:3 patients are suitable) or palliation with chemotherapy, radiotherapy, and/or a stenting tube. Tubes commonly become blocked. Good palliative care is essential—refer as necessary.

Prognosis:
- Overall—7% 5y survival (6% 10y survival)
- Surgical resection or radical chemoradiotherapy—10%–25% 5y survival
- Chemotherapy ± radiotherapy before surgery improves survival by ~13%.

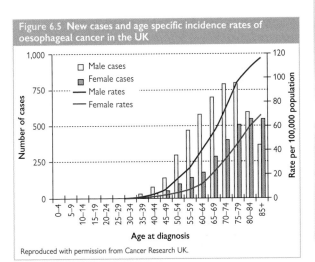

Figure 6.5 New cases and age specific incidence rates of oesophageal cancer in the UK

Reproduced with permission from Cancer Research UK.

Advice for patients

Looking after an oesophageal stent to prevent it from blocking:

- Don't rush and sit up straight when eating
- Have soft food in small mouthfuls and chew it well
- Drink a little during and after meals—fizzy drinks are helpful
- Don't tackle large lumps of food—cut them up small and chew well
- Spit out anything not chewed
- Mix food supplements such as Complan very thoroughly—dry powder will block the stent
- If you feel the stent is blocked stop eating, drink a little, and walk around a bit
- If the blockage persists for more than 3 hours ring your GP or contact the hospital where you were treated
- Clean the stent after eating with a drink of soda water or lemonade or use this mixture: 4oz sugar, 2oz cream of tartar, 2oz sodium bicarbonate—use one teaspoon of the mixture in a half glass of water
- Keep teeth and dentures in good order so that chewing is effective.

Foods to avoid:

- Green salads/raw vegetables
- Fried egg white
- Hard boiled egg
- Fruit skins and pith of grapefruit and orange
- Tough meat and gristle
- Nuts and dried fruits
- Fish with bones
- White bread, crusty bread, or toast
- Shredded or puffed wheat
- Hard chips and crisps.

Further information:

Oesophageal patients' association ▢ www.opa.org.uk

123

Stomach cancer: Causes ~5,500 deaths/y in the UK. Overall 95% are adenocarcinomas (which may be classified as 'intestinal' or 'diffuse'). Disease affecting older people with 90% diagnosed >55y—although peak age of diagnosis of early stage cancer is ~55y ♂ > ♀ (5:3). Incidence has halved over the past 30y in the UK probably due to improved diet.

Other risk factors include the following:

- Geography—common in Japan
- Blood group A
- *Heliobacter Pylori* infection (not clear if eradication ↓ risk)
- Atrophic gastritis
- Pernicious anaemia
- Smoking
- Adenomatous polyps
- Social class
- Previous partial gastrectomy.

Presentation:

- *History:* Often non-specific. Presents with dyspepsia; weight ↓; anorexia or early satiety; vomiting; dysphagia; anaemia and/or GI bleeding. Have a high index of suspicion in any patient >55y with recent-onset dyspepsia (within 1y) and/or other risk factors
- *Examination:* Usually normal until incurable. Look for epigastric mass, hepatomegaly, jaundice, ascites, enlarged supraclavicular LN (Virchow node), and acanthosis nigricans.

Management: If suspected refer for urgent endoscopy. In early stages total/partial gastrectomy may be curative. Chemotherapy before and after radical surgery improves cure-rate. As gastric tumours are very invasive and spread early, most present at a later stage. Overall 5y survival is 12%—Table 6.11. >90% of patients who survive 5y, survive long term.

❗ Gastric lymphomas and gastrointestinal stromal tumours (GISTs) behave differently to adenocarcinomas, have different management and prognosis, and are best dealt with by specialist teams in large centres.

Pancreatic cancer: Approximately 3% of all malignancies causing 8,000 deaths/y in the UK. 80% of cases occur in patients >60y. ♂ > ♀ (3:2).

Risk factors:

- Smoking—causes 25%–30% of pancreatic cancers in the UK Risk returns to non-smoker levels 10–20y after cessation
- Chronic pancreatitis—usually related to excess alcohol
- Type II DM —relative risk ≈1.8
- Obesity—↑ risk by 19%
- Genetic—5% pancreatic cancers are hereditary—characterized presentation aged <30y and +ve family history
- Occupation—cancer is ↑ among nickel workers, and workers exposed to insecticides, radiation, lead, iron, or chromium.

Tumour characteristics:

- The majority of pancreatic tumours develop in the exocrine part of the gland. Overall 95% of tumours are adenocarcinomas. Rarely tumours develop from the endocrine part—these have better prognosis
- 75% arise in the head of the pancreas, 15% from the body, and 10% from the tail. Tumours arising in the head of the pancreas tend to present earlier and are easier to remove.
- Spread to local LNs occurs early and metastatic spread to the peritoneum, liver and lungs is frequently found at presentation.

Table 6.11 Staging and prognosis of stomach adenocarcinoma

Staging

Tumour			Lymph nodes involved		Metastases	
TX	Primary tumour cannot be assessed.	NX	Regional LNs cannot be assessed.	MX	Cannot be assessed.
Tis	Carcinoma in situ.	N0	No.	M0	No distant metastases.
T1	Invasion of submucosa.	N1	1–6 regional LNs involved.	M1	Spread outside the affected lobe.
T2	Invasion of muscularis propria (a) or subserosa (b).	N2	7–15 regional LNs involved.		
T3	Penetration of serosa.	N3	>15 regional LNs involved.		
T4	Invasion of adjacent structures				

Prognosis

Stage	% of patients	TNM equivalent	5y survival (%)
0		Tis N0 M0	100
1	1	T1/2 N0 M0 or T1 N0/1 M0	70
2	6	T3 N0 M0 or T2 N1 M0 or T1 N2 M0	42
3	14	T2 N2 M0 or T3 N1/2 M0 or T4 N0 M0	20
4	80	T1–3 N3 M0 or T4 N1–3 M0 or any T/N M1	5

Advice for patients

Advice and support:

Cancer Research UK ☎ 0808 800 4040 🖥 www.cancerhelp.org.uk
Macmillan Cancer Support ☎ 0808 808 0000 🖥 www.macmillan.org.uk

Presentation: Non-specific with:
- Gradual deterioration in health or fatigue
- Anorexia or weight ↓
- Pain—epigastric ± radiation → back—may be relieved by sitting forward
- Obstructive jaundice
- Diarrhoea/steatorrhoea due to malabsorption
- Early satiety, dyspepsia, or nausea/vomiting—due to gastric outlet obstruction
- Pancreatitis
- New diabetes
- Spontaneous venous thrombosis.

Examination: Check for weight ↓, epigastric orleft upper quadrant mass, hepatomegaly, jaundice. If jaundice is present the gallbladder may be palpable as a small rounded mass beneath the liver.

Management: Refer for urgent surgical assessment. Diagnosis is confirmed using a combination of USS, CT, MRI, and/or endoscopic retrograde cholangiopancreatography (ERCP). The only potentially curative treatment for pancreatic cancer is surgery but <15% of patients are suitable for surgery at presentation. The operation of choice is a Whipple's procedure (pancreaticoduodenectomy). This is undertaken at a specialist centre. Surgery is associated with significant morbidity and has a mortality rate of 5%–15%.

Palliative treatment: Patients with locally advanced or metastatic disease may benefit from surgical bypass of common bile duct and/or duodenal obstruction. An alternative is a biliary stent. Some survival benefit may be gained from chemotherapy. Refer for palliative care support for symptom control early.

Prognosis:
- Surgical resection—5y survival 7%–25%—median survival 11–20mo. Those that survive 5y are likely to survive long term
- Irresectable locally advanced disease—median survival 6–11mo
- Metastatic disease—median survival 2–6mo.

Liver cancer: Hepatocellular cancer (HCC) is rare in the UK (100 new cases and 100 deaths/y) but the incidence is increasing due to steatohepatitis (fatty liver) associated with obesity and DM. Much more common in areas of the world where hepatitis B is endemic (e.g. China, India). Arises from regenerating nodules in a cirrhotic liver. *Peak age:* 60–70y. Intra- and extrahepatic spread is common and occurs early.

Presentation: In a patient with known cirrhosis:
- Fatigue
- Fever
- Anorexia and/or weight ↓
- Ascites
- Rapid deterioration in liver function
- Haemorrhage into the peritoneal cavity (often fatal)

- Budd Chiari syndrome (occlusion of the hepatic vein resulting in jaundice, epigastric pain, and shock)
- *Examination*—may reveal an abdominal mass, hepatomegaly ± an arterial bruit over the tumour.

Management: If suspected check αFP and refer for urgent assessment. αFP >500ng/ml in a patient with known cirrhosis is almost certainly diagnostic. The most important prognostic factors are the number and size of the liver lesions and the presence of vascular involvement. Overall 95% of patients with cirrhosis have disease, which is too extensive for curative surgery, or their severely compromised liver function makes radical surgery inappropriate. Approximately 50% of patients without cirrhosis have resectable tumours. Surgery may be combined with liver transplantation. Inoperable tumours may be treated with hepatic artery ligation or embolization. Tumours respond poorly to chemo- or radiotherapy, but new molecularly-targeted agents such as sorafenib have shown promise in clinical trials.

Overall prognosis:
- Patients with cirrhosis—median survival 3mo
- Patients without cirrhosis—median survival 1y.

Cholangiocarcinoma: Rare adenocarcinoma of the biliary tract. May be associated with UC. Typically presents in patients >60y with jaundice, right upper quadrant pain, and weight loss. The only effective treatment is surgery, but that is only possible in 10%–20% of patients. Selected fit patients with unresectable disease may be offered palliative chemotherapy or enrolment in a clinical trial.

Gallbladder cancer: Rare. ♀ > ♂. Gallstones are a predisposing factor. Typically presents in patients >40y with right upper quadrant pain, anorexia, weight ↓, and jaundice. Surgical resection offers the only hope of cure but disease is usually advanced at presentation. Selected fit patients with unresectable disease may be offered palliative chemotherapy or enrolment in a clinical trial.

Further information:
NICE Referral guidelines for suspected cancer (2005) ⌨ www.nice.org.uk
SIGN Management of oesophageal and gastric cancer (2006)
⌨ www.sign.ac.uk
Cancer Research UK ⌨ www.cancerresearchuk.org

Colorectal cancer

Colorectal cancer accounts for 13% of all cancers and 16,000 deaths every year in the UK. Each day in the UK there are 100 new diagnoses of colorectal cancer—two thirds arising in the colon and the remainder in the rectum. Lifetime risk of developing colorectal cancer is 1:18–20; 83% of tumours occur in patients >60y and >95% are adenocarcinomas.

Adenomatous polyps: Bowel cancers arise from these polyps over many years. All polyps are removed due to risk of malignant change. Follow-up surveillance with repeated colonoscopy may be necessary depending on the number of polyps and their size (>1cm diameter polyps are associated with higher risk of malignant change).

Protective and risk factors:

Geography: More common in the developed world—dietary factors are thought to be responsible for variations.

Lifestyle factors:
- *Obesity*—↑ risk by 15% if overweight and 30% if obese—effect is most marked in pre-menopausal women
- *Dietary factors*—diets with less red and processed meat, and more vegetables, fibre, fish, and milk are associated with ↓ risk
- *Alcohol*—↑ risk for heavy drinkers—especially if also low folate.

Medication history:
- *HRT*—risk ↓ by 20% if ever taken; ↓ by 30% if taking HRT currently
- *COC*—risk ↓ by 18% if ever taken
- *Statins*—risk is ↓ after 5y use.

Other medical history:
- *History of gallbladder disease and/or cholecystectomy*—50% ↑ in risk
- *Type II DM*—30% ↑ risk
- *UC or Crohn's disease*—↑ risk.

Family history: 📖 p.28

Bowel cancer screening: 📖 p.28

Presentation: May be found at bowel cancer screening (📖 p.28). Clinical presentations depend on the site involved (Figure 6.6):
- *Change in bowel habit:* diarrhoea ± mucus, constipation, or alternating diarrhoea and constipation, tenesmus
- *Intestinal obstruction:* pain, distension, absolute constipation ± vomiting. May be an acute, sudden event (20% of patients not detected by screening present with an acute obstruction) or gradually evolve
- *Rectal bleeding:* bright red rectal bleeding or +ve faecal occult blood test—60% rectal tumours. Rarely melaena if high tumour.
- *Perforation:* causing generalized peritonitis, or into an adjacent viscus (e.g. bladder) resulting in a fistula
- *Spread:* abdominal distension 2° to ascites, jaundice, rectal/pelvic pain
- *General effects:* weight ↓, anorexia, anaemia, malaise.

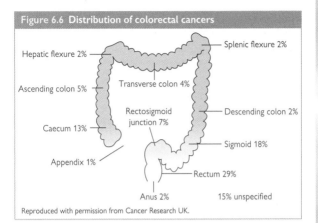

Figure 6.6 Distribution of colorectal cancers

Splenic flexure 2%
Hepatic flexure 2%
Transverse colon 4%
Ascending colon 5%
Rectosigmoid junction 7%
Descending colon 2%
Caecum 13%
Sigmoid 18%
Appendix 1%
Rectum 29%
Anus 2%
15% unspecified

Reproduced with permission from Cancer Research UK.

GMS contract			
Cancer 1	The practice can produce a register of all cancer patients defined as a 'register' of patients with a diagnosis of cancer excluding non-melanotic skin cancers from 1.4.2003.	5 points	
Cancer 3	% of patients with cancer, diagnosed within the last 18mo who have a patient review recorded as occurring within 6mo of the practice receiving confirmation of the diagnosis.	Up to 6 points	40%–90%
Education 7	The practice has undertaken a minimum of 12 significant event reviews in the past 3y which could include (if these have occurred) new cancer diagnoses.	Total of 4 points for 12 significant event reviews	

Advice for patients

Patient advice and support:
Macmillan Cancer Support ☎ 0808 808 0000
🖳 www.macmillan.org.uk
Colostomy Association ☎ 0800 328 4257
🖳 www.colostomyassociation.org.uk

Examination/investigation:

- General examination—cachexia, jaundice, anaemia
- Abdominal mass—palpable mass is present with 70% of right sided tumours and 40% of left sided tumours
- Hepatomegaly
- Ascites
- Rectal examination detects >75% of rectal tumours.
- FBC for anemia.

Management:

- Refer for urgent assessment (<2wk) to a colorectal surgeon
- Specialist confirmation of the diagnosis is with sigmoidoscopy/colonoscopy, barium enema and/or CT colography, and biopsy of the lesion
- If diagnosis is confirmed further investigations include liver function tests (LFTs), tumour markers (CEA is produced in >80% advanced tumours), CT of chest, abdomen and pelvis, and pelvic MRI for rectal cancers, to evaluate spread.

Treatment: Surgical resection is undertaken whenever possible. Pre-operative radiotherapy is often used in rectal cancer. Staging (Table 6.12) is based on findings at surgery and dictates further management with chemotherapy. Adjuvant chemotherapy ↓ risk of recurrence for high-risk node-negative and node-positive cases. For patients with more advanced disease, resection (with cure-rate of 30%) of or radioablation of hepatic metastases may be an option. Palliative chemotherapy has improved the average survival from 5–8mo to over 21mo.

Adverse pathological features	*Adverse clinical features*
• Presence and number of involved LNs	• Emergency presentation with bowel obstruction or perforation
• Lymphovascular, perineural, or venous invasion	• Incomplete resection
• Depth of penetration through bowel wall	• Metastatic disease
• Positive circumferential resection margin	• Presentation aged <50y.
• Mucinous histology	

Anal cancer: Usually squamous cell cancer (>50%).

Risk factors: Include anal sex; syphilis; anal warts (HPV).

Presentation: Bleeding, pain, anal mass, or ulcer, pruritus, stricture, change in bowel habit. A mass may be palpable on rectal examination. Check for inguinal LNs.

Management: Refer for urgent surgical review and confirmation of diagnosis. Treatment is usually with a combination of radiotherapy ± chemotherapy. AP resection is generally reserved for salvage therapy post-chemoradiotherapy failure.

Carcinoid tumours: Slow-growing tumours of low malignancy which arise from neuroendocrine cells or their precursors. *Incidence:* 3–4/100,000. *Peak age:* 61y. ♀ > ♂.

Sites:
- Intestinal—60% are in the midgut (especially appendix and terminal ileum)—examination may reveal an abdominal mass and/or enlarged liver. Rarely presents with bowel obstruction. Ileal carcinoids are multiple in 30%
- Non-intestinal—lung, testes, and ovary.

Carcinoid syndrome: This affects <10% of patients with a carcinoid tumour and develops when serotonin (5-HT) is released by the tumour and is not degraded by the liver due to hepatic metastases. Characteristic features:
- Paroxysmal flushing e.g. following alcohol or certain foods
- Watery, explosive diarrhoea
- Abdominal pain
- Bronchoconstriction—asthma-like reaction
- Right heart failure
- Rash—symmetrical, pruritic erythematous rash which blisters/crusts.

Management: refer for urgent assessment if suspected. Therapeutic options include somatostatin analogues such as octreotide or radiofrequency ablation of liver metastases. Prognosis—if no metastases the median survival is 5–8y; with metastases median survival is 38mo.

Table 6.12 Staging and prognosis of bowel cancer				
Stage	Modified Duke stage	Features and TNM equivalent	5y survival (%)
Stage 0	A (11% patients)	Carcinoma *in situ*.	83
Stage I		No LNs affected. No distant metastases. Tumour invades submucosa (T1 N0 M0). Tumour invades muscularis propria (T2 N0 M0).	
Stage II	B (35% patients)	No LNs affected. No distant metastases. Tumour invades subserosa (T3 N0 M0). Tumour invades other organs (T4 N0 M0).	64
Stage III	C (26% patients)	No distant metastases. 1–3 LNs involved (any T N1 M0). ≥4 LNs involved (any T N2 M0).	38
Stage IV	D (29% patients)	Distant metastases (any T any N M1).	3

Further information:

NICE Referral guidelines for suspected cancer—quick reference guide (2005) ⌨ www.nice.org.uk
NHS Bowel Cancer Screening Programme
⌨ www.cancerscreening.nhs.uk
SIGN Management of colorectal cancer (2003) ⌨ www.sign.ac.uk
Adjuvant online—decision making tool for professionals. assessing risks and benefits of additional therapy after surgery ⌨ www.adjuvantonline.com

Acute leukaemia

Clonal malignant disorders (from a single cell) affecting all age groups.

Acute lymphoblastic leukaemia (ALL): The abnormal proliferation is in the lymphoid progenitor cells (Figure 6.7). Incidence is 1–4/100,000 population/y. ♂ > ♀. The usual age range is 2–10y with a peak at 3–4y. Accounts for 85% of childhood leukaemia. Incidence then falls with increasing age apart from a secondary peak at ~40y.

Acute myeloid leukaemia (AML): Derived from abnormal proliferation of a myeloid progenitor cell (Figure 6.7). There are at least seven different subtypes. This is the most common leukaemia of adulthood with incidence of ~1.5/100,000 population/y. Incidence ↑ with age. Median age at presentation is ≈60y. ♂ = ♀. Risk factors include smoking (1:5 cases); previous chemotherapy or radiotherapy and exposure to radiation. Children with Down's syndrome are more likely to develop AML.

Presentation: Short history (weeks). Symptoms/signs arise from:
Bone marrow failure:
- Anaemia—pallor, lethargy, dyspnoea
- Neutropenia—infections of the mouth, throat, skin, fever
- Thrombocytopenia—spontaneous bruising, menorrhagia, bleeding from wounds, bleeding of gums, or nose bleeds.

Organ infiltration:
- Superficial lymphadenopathy (>50%)
- Hepatosplenomegaly (70%)
- Bone pain (ALL only)
- Skin infiltration (AML only)
- Testicular enlargement
- Respiratory symptoms due to mediastinal LNs
- Gum hypertrophy
- Unexplained irritability/behaviour change/drop in performance.

Differential diagnosis:
- Infections e.g. Epstein–Barr virus
- Other blood conditions e.g. aplastic anaemia, ITP, myelodysplasia
- Other malignancies e.g. lymphoma, neuroblastoma, metastatic disease
- Rheumatoid arthritis.

Investigation:
- *FBC:* normal or ↓ Hb and platelets; WCC <1×10^9/l to >200×10^9/l.
- *Blood film:* is abnormal with presence of blast cells
- *U&E:* renal impairment if leukocyte count is very high
- *CXR* may show mediastinal mass and/or lytic bone lesions.

Initial management: Refer for same-day haematology or paediatric opinion if:
- Abnormal blood count reported as needing urgent investigation
- Petechiae/pupura/spontaneous bleeding
- Fatigue in a previously healthy individual if accompanied by generalized lymphadenopathy and/or hepatosplenomegaly
- Any other suspicious symptoms/signs.

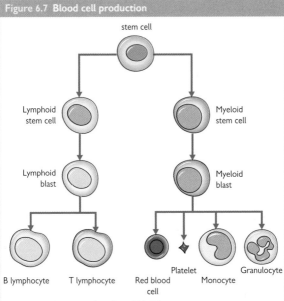

Figure 6.7 Blood cell production

stem cell

Lymphoid stem cell — Myeloid stem cell

Lymphoid blast — Myeloid blast

B lymphocyte — T lymphocyte — Red blood cell — Platelet — Monocyte — Granulocyte

Reproduced with permission from Cancer Help UK.

GMS contract

Cancer 1	The practice can produce a register of all cancer patients defined as a 'register' of patients with a diagnosis of cancer excluding non-melanotic skin cancers from 1.4.2003.	5 points	
Cancer 3	% of patients with cancer, diagnosed within the last 18mo who have a patient review recorded as occurring within 6mo of the practice receiving confirmation of the diagnosis.	Up to 6 points	40%–90%
Education 7	The practice has undertaken a minimum of 12 significant event reviews in the past 3y which could include (if these have occurred) new cancer diagnoses.	Total of 4 points for 12 significant event reviews	

Specialist management: Confirmation of the diagnosis is made by examining a bone marrow smear and performing appropriate cyto-chemical, immunocytochemical, and cytogenetic examinations, and flow cytometry. Treatment is co-ordinated in specialized centres and involves intensive supportive care together with systemic chemotherapy and radiotherapy ± bone marrow transplant.

Phases of treatment:
- *Remission induction*—aims to remove leukaemia cells from the blood/bone marrow—involves chemotherapy (in all cases) ± steroids (ALL) ± radiotherapy (ALL). Growth factors may be given after chemotherapy to aid recovery of normal bone marrow
- *Consolidation/intensification*—aims to stop recurrence following remission—involves chemotherapy ± autologous stem cell or donor bone marrow/stem cell transplant
- *Maintenance*—Chemotherapy + steroids—given to ALL patients for up to 2y to help maintain remission
- *Prophylactic treatment*—intra-thecal chemotherapy or radiotherapy is given to patients with ALL to prevent spread to the brain/spine.

Short-term side effects of treatment:
- *Treatment side effects:* Most chemotherapeutic agents have pronounced side effects e.g. nausea, vomiting, hair loss, neuropathy
- *Immunosuppression:* Any fever in a neutropenic child or adult must be taken seriously and referred immediately back to the unit in charge of care. Likewise any chickenpox contact must be referred immediately for consideration of administration of zoster Ig, or measles contact for administration of measles Ig.

Long-term side effects of treatment:
- Heart—cardiomyopathy, arrhythmias
- Lung—fibrosis
- Endocrine system—growth delay, hypothyroidism, infertility
- Kidney—↓ glomerular filtration rate
- Secondary malignancies—may appear after many years
- Psychological effects.

Prognosis: See Tables 6.13 and 6.14.

Table 6.13 Prognosis of acute leukaemia	
Type	**Overall 5y survival (%)**
Childhood ALL	65–75
Adult ALL	40 (80 achieve remission)
AML age <55y	40–60
AML age >55y	20

Further information:
NICE Referral guidelines for suspected cancer (2005) ⌨ www.nice.org.uk

Table 6.14 Prognostic factors

AML	ALL
Age—poorer prognosis with ↑ age.	Age—prognosis is better the younger the patient (excluding children <2y).
WCC at diagnosis—poorer prognosis the higher the WCC.	Gender—females do better than males.
Past medical history—myelodysplasia or treatment for another cancer results in poorer prognosis.	Race—Caucasians have better prognosis.
Cytogenetics of leukaemia cells—balanced translocations confer good prognosis; complex karyotypes confer poor prognosis.	WCC at diagnosis—poorer prognosis the higher the WCC.
	CNS involvement at diagnosis has poorer prognosis.
	Type of white cell affected.
Time taken to get the disease under control—good prognosis if under control in one or two cycles of chemotherapy.	Cytogenetics of leukaemia cells.
	Time taken to achieve remission—if <4wk then better prognosis; if leukaemia cells still present when induction is complete then poorer prognosis.

GP notes

Bone marrow investigation:

- Samples are usually taken from the posterior iliac crest using local anaesthetic
- Usually bone marrow is aspirated and also a core of bone marrow is removed (trephine)
- The trephine biopsy is particularly useful in those cases in which no bone marrow can be aspirated (dry tap) or if only blood is aspirated (blood tap)
- Patients with low platelet counts may require platelet transfusion before the procedure to prevent bruising/bleeding.

Advice for patients

Information and support:

Leukaemia Care ☎ 0800 169 6680 🖳 www.leukaemiacare.org
Leukaemia Society 🖳 www.leukaemiasociety.org
Leukaemia and Lymphoma Research 🖳 www.llresearch.org.uk
Children with Leukaemia ☎ 020 7404 0808
🖳 www.leukaemia.org.uk
CLIC and Sargent ☎ 0800 197 0068 🖳 www.clicsargent.org.uk

Lymphoma

Lymphoma is cancer of the lymphatic system. There are two main types.

Non-Hodgkin's lymphoma (NHL): Derived from malignant transformation of lymphocytes—B cells in most cases (85%). Usually develops in lymph nodes but can arise in any other tissue (25%–30%). Most common extra-nodal sites are the stomach, skin, and small intestine.

Incidence: 10,500 cases/y in the UK (4% cancers), causing 4,500 deaths/y. ♂ = ♀. 69% occur in patients >60y. Incidence has ↑ by 6% in the past 10y (Table 6.15).

Classification: There are many different types of NHL. The World Health Organization (WHO) classification divides NHL into categories based on:
- Grade—aggressive (high grade) or non-aggressive (indolent/low grade)
- Type of cell involved—T cell, B cell, or unknown cell (null/killer cell)
- Appearance under the microscope—large cell or small cell and follicular (grouped) or diffuse.

Risk factors:
- *Age*—incidence ↑ with age
- *Infection*—EBV is linked with Burkitt's lymphoma; *Helicobacter pylori* infection with primary gastric lymphoma, and *Chlamydia psittaci* infection with orbital lymphoma
- *Immune suppression*—transplant patients have ↑ risk—13% heart transplant and 33% heart/lung transplant patients develop NHL; HIV/AIDS patients have a 15× ↑ risk of low grade and 400× ↑ risk of high-grade NHL (although only 3%–5% develop NHL)
- *Genetic*—familial clusters of NHL do occur. May also be associated with genetic conditions e.g. ataxia telangectasia (↑ B cell lymphoma) and genetically determined immunodeficiency states (e.g. common variable hypogammalobulinaemia)
- *Coeliac disease*—associated with intestinal T cell lymphoma
- *Inflammation*—associated with Hashimoto's thyroiditis; patients with rheumatoid arthritis and Sjögren's syndrome have ↑ risk.

Presentation: May be detected incidentally on CXR (mediastinal mass) or present with:
- Painless peripheral lymphadenopathy
- Abdominal mass (nodal or spleen)
- Weight ↓
- Night sweats/unexplained fevers.

Other symptoms are dependent on site e.g. neurological symptoms if CNS involvement; pleural effusion; skin lesions.

Investigation:
- *FBC:* may be normal if no bone marrow involvement
- *Monospot:* perform in all patients <30y with persistent lymphadenopathy to exclude Epstein-Barr Virus
- *ESR:* usually ↑
- *Liver function tests:* abnormal if liver involvement.

Table 6.15 Features of common types of NHL

Type	Features
High-grade NHL	
Diffuse large B cell (DLBCL)	20% of NHL (including childhood). For adults peak age = 70y. Presents with rapidly enlarging lymphadenopathy. Extra-nodal involvement is common. 10% have bone marrow involvement at presentation.
Anaplastic large cell	Two forms. Both originate from T cells or unknown cells. *Systemic form:* affects children/young adults. ♀ > ♂. Usually presents at a late stage and with systemic symptoms. *Cutaneous form:* 5% NHL. Affects adults (peak age 61y). Presents with reddish brown skin nodules or ulceration ± regional LN involvement (25%).
Burkitt's	Affects children—30%–40% childhood lymphoma. ♂ > ♀. B cell lymphoma. Two varieties—endemic variety is more common in Africa and associated with Epstein-Barr virus infection. Peak age 5–10y; sporadic variety occurs worldwide and affects slightly older children. Presents with bulky central nodal disease ± extra-nodal (typically abdomen), bone marrow and/or CNS involvement.
Low-grade NHL	
Follicular	Affects adults. B cell origin. Three types divided according to the ratio of small and large cells. Usually presents with disseminated disease. 50% with bone marrow involvement. May transform to DLBCL.
Small lymphocytic	4–5% NHL. Median age 60y. Clinically/morphologically identical to CLL (🕮 p.140). Distinguished by the degree of lymph tissue vs. blood/bone marrow involvement. Presents with diffuse lymphadenopathy and some blood/bone marrow involvement. 10%–20% transform to CLL, 3% to DLBCL.
Mantle cell	5% NHL. Affects adults usually >50y. ♂ > ♀ (4:1). Although classified as low grade, behaves and is treated as high grade. Usually presents with widespread disease involving LNs, bone marrow (60%–90%), peripheral blood and spleen. Poor prognosis.
Marginal zone	B-cell origin. Three distinct types: *Nodal:* 1%–3% NHL. Presents with localized lymphadenopathy. *Splenic:* <1% NHL. Affects adults. Presents with massive splenomegaly and blood/bone marrow involvement without lymphadenopathy. *Mucosa associated (MALT):* 10% NHL. May be associated with inflammation (e.g. *H. pylori* infection and gastric MALT; Hashimoto's thyroiditis and thyroid MALT). 70% have localized disease on presentation. Symptoms depend on the organ involved.
Lympho-plasmacytic	1.5% NHL. Also called Waldenstrom's macroglobulinaemia. B cell lymphoma. Average age at presentation is 63y. Often presents late with lymphadenopathy, splenomegaly, and bone marrow involvement. May spread to the lung or GI tract. Usually associated with paraproteinaemia (IgM).

Initial management: Consider discussion with a haematologist, urgent referral for LN biopsy, or urgent referral to haematology if:
- Lymphadenopathy present ≥6wk
- LNs are increasing in size or LN >2cm in size
- Widespread lymphadenopathy
- Lymphadenopathy + weight ↓, night sweats and/or splenomegaly
- Any other suspicious symptoms/signs.

Specialist treatment: It is based on histology and stage (Table 6.16). Strategies broadly divide into those for whom disease is:
- *Limited*—tumours <10cm diameter; stage 1/2 disease; no B symptoms
- *Advanced*—tumour >10cm diameter; stage 3/4 disease; B symptoms.

Treatment options include:
- *Wait and see*—may be used for low-grade lymphomas
- *Radiotherapy*—disease restricted to one LN group and CNS lymphoma; for other lymphomas may be used to treat local disease in combination with chemotherapy
- *Chemotherapy*—single agent or combination (e.g. CHOP; cyclophosphamide, hydroxydaunorubicin [doxorubicin; Adriamycin®], Oncovin® [vincristine], and prednisone/prednisolone); intensive chemotherapy + autologous stem cell transplant may be used to treat some recurrent lymphomas (e.g. large cell or follicular NHL)
- *Other*—monoclonal antibody treatment (e.g. rituximab which targets B-cells) is widely used ± chemotherapy; trials of immunotherapy (vaccines, allotransplantation) show promising results. In gastric MALT, eradication of *H. pylori* may induce remission. Anti-viral agents may be useful in Epstein-Barr virus-related NHL.

Prognosis: Varies widely between different types of NHL and the age of the patient (Box 6.1). Overall 5y survival is 51% with 45% surviving 10y.

Hodgkin's lymphoma: Approximately 1,200 cases/y. occur in the UK. *Peak age ranges:* 15–35y (>50% occur <40y) and 50–70y. These are derived from B lymphocytes. Two types are recognized:
- *Classical* (95%)—Reed Sternberg cells present. Subdivides into nodular sclerozing (>50% of all Hodgkin's lymphoma), mixed cellularity, lymphocyte depleting, and lymphocyte rich types
- *Nodular lymphocyte predominant* (5%) -'Popcorn' cells present.

Presentation: Painless lymphadenopathy (95%—70% have affected cervical LNs at diagnosis), weight ↓, night sweats/unexplained fevers, pruritus. The spleen is involved in 30% → splenomegaly.

Investigation and initial management: Similar to that for NHL.

Specialist treatment: Depends mainly on stage of disease:
- Stages 1–2A—chemotherapy + radiotherapy to affected LNs ± spleen
- Stages 2B–4—chemotherapy ± steroids ± radiotherapy
- Relapse—may be treated with intensive chemotherapy + stem cell transplant.

Prognosis:
- *Early stage disease* (Ann Arbor stage 1 or 2—affected lymph tissue is confined to one side of the diaphragm)—80% 10y survival
- *Late-stage disease* (Ann Arbor stage 3 or 4—affected lymph tissue both sides of diaphragm and/or extra-lymphatic tissue involvement)—60% 5y survival.

Table 6.16 The simplified Ann Arbor system of staging lymphoma

Stage	Definition
1	Involvement of single LN region or lymphoid structure (e.g. spleen).
2	Involvement of ≥2 LN regions/structures on the same side of the diaphragm.
3	Involvement of LN regions/structures on both sides of the diaphragm.
4	Involvement of extra-nodal sites e.g. liver, bone marrow. Classified as stage 4E if only one extra-nodal site.

Further subdivision of stages:

A	No symptoms.
B	Fever >38°C; drenching sweats; weight loss (>10% in 6mo).

Box 6.1 Prognostic index for NHL

Score 1 point for each of the following:
- Age >60y
- Stage 3 or 4 at diagnosis
- Serum lactate dehydrogenase (LDH) levels
- Performance status >2 (in bed/chair for >50% of each day and needs help with activities of daily living)
- NHL in >one extra-nodal site.

Score 1 or 2—good prognosis
Score 3—moderately high risk of lack of treatment response/recurrence
Score 4 or 5—high risk of lack of treatment response/recurrence.

GMS contract

Cancer 1	The practice can produce a register of all cancer patients defined as a 'register' of patients with a diagnosis of cancer excluding non-melanotic skin cancers from 1.4.2003.	5 points	
Cancer 3	% of patients with cancer, diagnosed within the last 18mo who have a patient review recorded as occurring within 6mo of the practice receiving confirmation of the diagnosis.	Up to 6 points	40%–90%
Education 7	The practice has undertaken a minimum of 12 significant event reviews in the past 3y which could include (if these have occurred) new cancer diagnoses.	Total of 4 points for 12 significant event reviews	

Advice for patients

Information and support:
Lymphoma Association ☎ 0808 808 5555 🖳 www.lymphomas.org.uk

Other haematological malignancies

Chronic lymphocytic leukaemia (CLL): Occurs in the elderly accounting for 40% leukaemias in that age group. CLL is closely related to small lymphocytic lymphoma (📖 p.137).

Presentation: Widespread painless lymphadenopathy often noted over a period of months/years. *Examination:* Lymphadenopathy, spleno- ± hepatomegaly.

Investigation: 70%–80% all diagnoses follow FBC done for another reason—↑ WCC (>30 × 10^9/L). Blood film—small lymphocytes—many of which are disrupted to form characteristic 'smear' cells.

Management: Refer urgently to haematology. Treatment is determined by Binet stage of disease:
- A—high WCC, ≤3 groups of involved LNs
- B—high WCC, >3 groups of involved LNs
- C—high WCC and low red cell and platelet counts; involvement of LNs or spleen.

⓵ A group is defined as LNs in one area of the body (e.g. cervical). Where bilateral LNs are involved (e.g. groin), it counts as a single group.

Treatment is often unnecessary for early, symptomless CLL due to the benign nature of the disease and age group it affects. Later stage disease in younger patients and/or symptomatic disease may require chemotherapy and/or radiotherapy. Prognosis is generally good with many surviving >10y.

Chronic myeloid (granulocytic) leukaemia: *Peak age:* 30–60y.

Presentation: Found by chance in 20% patients. Otherwise presents with non-specific symptoms e.g. weight ↓, lassitude, gout, anaemia. Splenomegaly is common and the spleen may be so enlarged that patients present with abdominal pain, digestive symptoms, or pleuritic pain due to splenic infarction. Rarely abnormal bleeding occurs due to abnormal platelet function.

Investigation: *FBC:* ↑ WCC (usually >50 × 10^9/l) ± anaemia. *Blood film:* bone marrow precursors of myeloid cells (blasts).

Management: Refer urgently to haematology. Treatment is determined by phase of the disease:
- *Chronic* (90% at diagnosis)—<10% of cells in the bone marrow are immature blasts. Treatment of choice is imatinib (Glivec®)
- *Accelerated*—10%–30% of cells in the bone marrow are immature blasts. Treatment is with chemotherapy or dasatinib (unless not previously treated with imatinib). Intensive chemotherapy + bone marrow or stem cell transplant is an option
- *Blast* (also called acute phase, blast crisis)—>30% of cells in the bone marrow are immature blasts—treated with chemotherapy.

Prognosis: Median survival was 3–4y from diagnosis but the recent introduction of imatinib is likely to improve prognosis considerably.

Myeloproliferative disorders: proliferation of ≥1 of the haemopoi-
etic components of the bone marrow. Includes the following:
● Chronic myeloid leukaemia (see opposite page)
● Primary proliferative polycythaemia (see below)
● Essential thrombocythaemia (see below)
● Myelofibrosis (see below).

Primary proliferative polycythaemia (PPP): Also known as
polycythaemia rubra vera and erythrocytosis. Haematological malignancy resulting in overproduction of red cells. *Age range:* most >50y.

Presentation: Non-specific symptoms/signs:
● Night sweats
● Dusky, cyanotic hue with red-face
● Itching (especially provoked by water e.g. after a bath)
● Headaches, dizziness, vertigo, and/or tinnitus
● Gout—due to high red cell turnover
● Thrombosis and haemorrhage—due to abnormal platelet function
  and hyperviscosity
● Peptic ulceration (5%–10%)
● Splenomegaly (70%) ± hepatomegaly.

Investigation: May be diagnosed incidentally following FBC done for
other reasons—↑ Hb (usually >20g/dL) + haematocrit (>0.52 for ♂;
>0.48 for ♀) sustained for >2mo.

Differential diagnosis:
● Compensatory polycythaemia e.g. smoking, COPD, cyanotic heart
  disease, high-altitude living
● Haemoconcentration e.g. due to dehydration or plasma loss
● Renal disease
● Other haematological conditions e.g. methaemoglobinaemia
● Other malignancy e.g. hepatocellular, renal.

Management: Refer urgently to haematology. Patients remain at risk
from thrombosis and haemorrhage unless the Hb level is ↓ by regular
venesection. Oral hydroxyurea chemotherapy is an option. The disease
is slowly progressive and survival for 10–20y is not unusual—10%–20%
eventually transform to acute leukaemia; 1:3 to myelofibrosis.

Essential thrombocythaemia: Rare disorder. Patients have ↑ risk
of both thrombosis and haemorrhage due to abnormal platelet function. *FBC*—Platelet count is persistently >600 × 10^9/l.; WCC is normal
or ↑; Hb is ↑ or ↓. Refer urgently to haematology. Treatment is usually
with hydroxyurea or interferon. May eventually transform to acute
leukaemia.

Myelofibrosis (myelosclerosis): Progressive accumulation of
fibrous tissue in the bone marrow cavity replacing normal marrow.
Haemopoietic function is taken over by the spleen and liver.

Presentation: Patients are usually elderly and present with symptoms of
anaemia, malaise, fever ± gout. The spleen is massively enlarged.

Investigation: FBC—↓ Hb; *Blood film*—immature erythroid cells (nor-
moblasts) and myeloid cells (metamyelocytes/myelocytes). Red cells
are tear-drop shaped.

Management: Refer urgently to haematology. Treatment is generally unsatisfactory though some patients may be given chemotherapy to improve white cell/platelet counts or constitutional symptoms. Splenectomy may help but is high risk. Median survival is 2–3y—but many live much longer. May transform to acute leukaemia.

Myelodysplastic syndromes: Comprise a group of disorders characterized by ineffective production of ≥1 haemopoietic cell line. Differs from myeloproliferative disorder as there is no invasion of normal marrow by abnormal cells. Affects elderly patients and may be discovered incidentally or present with anaemia and/or bleeding. The spleen may be palpable but is never grossly enlarged. FBC and blood film are diagnostic. Refer urgently to haematology—treatment is with transfusion and prompt treatment of infection ± chemotherapy. Tends to evolve gradually to acute myeloid leukaemia (75% in <2y).

Multiple myeloma: *Age:* Usually >50y. 4,000 new cases/y in the UK and 2,700 deaths. A mutant B lymphoid clone is present. The proliferating cells grow mainly in the bone marrow where they cause infiltration, localized tumours, and bone erosion. Main sites of myeloma involvement are: skull, spinal column, thoracic cage, pelvis, and proximal long bones.

Presentation:
- Infection e.g. chest infection
- Anaemia
- Bone pain ± tenderness— particularly back, pelvis or femur
- Pathological fracture
- Hypercalcaemia
- Renal failure
- Hyperviscosity syndrome (CNS features e.g. blurred vision, altered consciousness, confusion)
- Amyloidosis (heart, tongue, carpal tunnel).

Investigation:
- *FBC*—anaemia; *blood film*—rouleaux formation
- *ESR* ↑↑
- *Renal function:* ↑ Cr; ↓ eGFR
- *Ca^{2+}:* frequently ↑
- *Serum electrophoresis:* paraprotein band
- *Urine electrophoresis:* Bence Jones protein
- *X-ray:* erosive lesions in skull, ribs, pelvis. Fractures and vertebral collapse are common.

⚠ Some patients have a paraprotein band in isolation with no other features of myeloma (monoclonal gammopathy of uncertain significance—MGUS). The M-protein level may remain unchanged for many years or slowly progress to myeloma.

Management: Refer urgently to haematology. Specialist management depends on symptoms and whether there is tissue/organ damage.
- *Asymptomatic disease*—patients are usually monitored closely and treatment starts if symptoms or tissue/organ damage develop

- *Symptomatic disease*—Treatment is with melphalan or combination chemotherapy, and steroids. A new generation of biological agents (bortezomib and lenalidomide) has significantly prolonged the effects of chemotherapy. Bisphosphonates are used to prevent and treat hypercalcaemia and bone pain. Bone pain may also respond to radiotherapy. Renal failure may require dialysis. Hyperviscosity may require plasmapheresis. Intensive chemotherapy and bone marrow or stem cell transplant is an option for younger, fit patients
- *Relapsed disease*—patients who have gone into remission almost always relapse at some point. If relapse is >6mo after initial treatment the patient is usually retreated with the same chemotherapy. Otherwise an alternative regime is used. Again, the role of lenalidomide, bortezomib, and other novel agents in treatment of relapse is under evaluation.

Prognosis: Overall 5y survival is 23%. However, for patients <70y who are fit enough to undergo intensive treatment, 5y survival more than doubles to 50%.

GMS contract			
Cancer 1	The practice can produce a register of all cancer patients defined as a 'register' of patients with a diagnosis of cancer excluding non-melanotic skin cancers from 1.4.2003.	5 points	
Cancer 3	% of patients with cancer, diagnosed within the last 18mo who have a patient review recorded as occurring within 6mo of the practice receiving confirmation of the diagnosis.	Up to 6 points	40%–90%
Education 7	The practice has undertaken a minimum of 12 significant event reviews in the past 3y which could include (if these have occurred) new cancer diagnoses.	Total of 4 points for 12 significant event reviews	

Brain and spinal cord tumours

Brain tumours are relatively rare. There are 4,500 new cases of primary brain or spinal cord cancer diagnosed each year in the UK and the average GP will see approximately four new cases of brain tumour in a career. Peak age of diagnosis is 70–74y but brain tumour is the most common childhood cancer affecting 300 children/y in the UK.

Secondary brain tumours: 30% of clinical brain tumours are due to metastatic spread of tumour from elsewhere in the body—usually breast, lung, kidney, bowel, or melanoma. In 50%, brain metastases are multiple. As patients live longer with metastatic cancer due to improved therapies, brain metastases are increasingly seen.

Primary CNS tumours: Classified according to grade and cell type (Table 6.17). Tumours are graded 1–4 histologically. Although primary CNS tumours almost never metastasize outside the CNS, low-grade tumours (grade 1 and 2) tend to be less aggressive than high-grade tumours (grade 3 and 4).

Risk factors:

- Genetic—5% are associated with known genetic conditions e.g. neurofibromatosis, tuberous sclerosis, Li-Fraumeni, or Von Hippel–Lindau syndrome
- Previous cranial radiotherapy—e.g. for childhood ALL
- Weakened immunity—associated with cerebral lymphoma
- Cerebral palsy.

🖋 There is no proven link between mobile phone use and brain tumours

Presentation of intra-cranial tumours:

- ↑ *ICP:* Papilloedema 23%–50% at presentation; headache 25%–35%
- *Seizures:* 25%–30%. Suspect in all adults who have a first seizure. Refer for urgent neurological assessment
- *Evolving focal neurology:* Depends on the site. >50% have focal neurology at presentation. Frontal lobe lesions tend to present late
- *False localizing signs:* Caused by ↑ ICP. VI nerve palsy (causing double vision) is most common due to its long intracranial course
- *Subtle personality change:* 16%–20% at presentation—irritability, lack of application, lack of initiative, socially inappropriate behaviour
- *Local effects:* Skull base masses, proptosis, epistaxis.

⚠ <1% of patients presenting with headache have a brain tumour.

Differential diagnosis:

Other space occupying lesions—aneurysm, abscess, chronic subdural haematoma, granuloma, cyst.

- Stroke
- Multiple sclerosis
- Head injury
- Vasculitis
- Encephalitis
- Todds palsy
- Metabolic or electrolyte disturbance.

Action: If suspected, depending on clinical state, admit as an acute medical emergency or refer for urgent neurological assessment.

Treatment: Surgery (depending on the site and extent of the tumour) ± radiotherapy. After surgical resection, patients with recurrent glioma and good performance status may be offered combination radiotherapy + chemotherapy with temozolomide. Other chemotherapy may be used for cerebral lymphoma, and some brain secondaries.

Prognosis: Prognosis depends on: tumour type, grade, and site; symptoms at presentation; and, age of the patient. Overall there is a 30% 1y and 14% 5y survival.

Table 6.17 Types of primary CNS tumour	
Type	**Notes**
Glioma Subtypes include	50% of all primary brain tumours—umbrella term for tumours of nervous system origin.
• Astrocytoma	80% gliomas—grade 3 astrocytoma (anaplastic astrocytoma) and grade 4 astrocytoma (glioblastoma multi-form) are the most common forms of brain tumour in adults.
• Oligodendroglioma	10%–15% gliomas.
• Ependymoma	5% gliomas.
• Mixed	
Meningioma	25% of brain tumours in adults—arise from meninges—usually found in the forebrain or hindbrain and grow slowly. Rarely associated with neurofibromatosis type 2.
Medulloblastoma	Medulloblastoma—primitive neuroectodermal tumour—usually found in the cerebellum. 70% occur in children (accounts for 25% brain tumours in children—peak age 3–5y) but can also occur in adults.
Pituitary adenoma	10% of brain tumours—usually benign and often present with endocrine signs/symptoms due to over production or lack of pituitary hormones.
Craniopharyngioma	Base of the brain—usually affect children, teenagers or young adults.
Haemangioblastoma	2% of brain tumours—arise from blood vessels. May be associated with von Hippel–Lindau syndrome.
Acoustic neuroma	More common in older adults—may present with unilateral deafness—may be associated with neurofibromatosis type 2.
Pineal tumour	1% brain tumours—may release αFP and/or HCG tumour markers.
Cerebral lymphoma	Associated with immunosuppression e.g. HIV
Spinal cord tumours	20% of CNS tumours are in the spine. Usually neurofibromas or meningiomas; rarely chordomas, Schwannomas, or neuroblastomas.

145

Advice for patients

Support for patients and carers:
Brain Tumour UK ☎ 0845 4500 386 🖳 www.braintumouruk.org.uk
Brain and spine foundation ☎ 0808 808 1000
🖳 www.brainandspine.org.uk

Skin cancer

Prevention of skin cancer: 📖 p.17

Basal cell carcinoma (rodent ulcer, BCC): Accounts for >75% of skin cancer in the UK but is almost never fatal. Locally invasive but rarely metastasizes. Tends to occur in middle aged/elderly patients, may be multiple and appears mainly on light-exposed areas—especially the face.

Major types: There are three main types (all can be pigmented):
- *Nodular*—most common—starts as a small pearly nodule which may necrose centrally leaving a small crusted ulcer with a pearly, rolled edge—Figure 6.8
- *Cystic*
- *Multi-centric*—plaque-like, large, superficial ± central depression.

Causes:
- Sun exposure
- X-ray irradiation
- Chronic scarring
- Genetic predisposition
- Arsenic ingestion.

Management: Complete excision is ideal. Alternatives are radiotherapy (>60y), photodynamic therapy, cryotherapy, curettage, and cautery. Refer to dermatology, general surgery, plastic surgery, or radiotherapy as appropriate.

Prognosis: Recurrence rate is 5% at 5y for all modalities of treatment. Development of new BCC at other sites is common.

Squamous cell carcinoma (SCC): 20% of skin cancer in the UK. Most common in patients aged > 55y. ♂ > ♀. May metastasize (10%). Usually develops in light-exposed sites e.g. face, neck, hands. May start within an actinic (solar) keratosis or *de novo* as a nodule which progresses to ulcerate and form a crust—Figure 6.9.

Causes:
- Chronic sun damage
- X-ray exposure
- Chronic ulceration and scarring (aggressive SCC may develop at the edge of chronic ulcers)
- Smoking pipes and cigars (lip lesions)
- Industrial carcinogens (tars, oils)
- Wart virus
- Immunosuppression
- Genetic.

Management: Refer to dermatology. Treated with surgical excision ± LN biopsy. Large lesions may require skin grafting. Radiotherapy is an alternative for large lesions in elderly patients.

Bowen's disease: Intraepidermal carcinoma. Common—typically on the lower leg in elderly women. Lesions are pink/slightly pigmented scaly plaques (<5cm diameter) and may be solitary or multiple—Figure 6.10. *Risk factor:* exposure to arsenicals. Transformation to SCC is rare.

Management: Biopsy confirms diagnosis. Treatment is with cryotherapy, curettage, or excision.

Figure 6.8 Basal cell carcinoma on lower eyelid

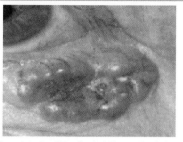

Reproduced with permission from ⬚ http://medweb.bham.ac.uk/easdec/eyetextbook/
CA-%20Eye/Ca-eye.htm

Figure 6.9 Squamous cell carcinoma on the dorsum of a hand

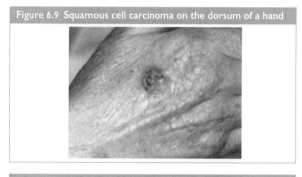

Figure 6.10 Bowen's disease

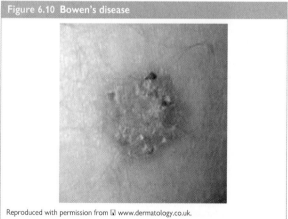

Reproduced with permission from ⬚ www.dermatology.co.uk.

147

Cutaneous malignant melanoma: Cancer usually starting in the skin, either in a mole or in normal-looking skin. The number of people who develop melanoma is rising in the UK. At present there are ≈10,400 new cases/y in the UK, ♀:♂ ≈ 2:1, and 2,700 deaths. It occurs in all races although is particularly common in fair-skinned Caucasians. Overall 10% have a family history. Frequently metastasizes—may present with metastasis.

Major types of skin melanoma: Figure 6.11
- *Superficial spreading:* 70% UK cases. ♀ > ♂. usually presents in middle age. *Most common site:* lower leg in ♀ (50%); back in ♂. Macular lesion with variable pigmentation. Initially spreads across the surface of the skin before invading deeper
- *Nodular:* ♂ > ♀. 20% UK cases. Most common on the trunk. Pigmented nodule grows rapidly and may ulcerate
- *Lentigo:* A lentigo maligna arises in sun-damaged skin—most common on the face—and melanoma develops many years afterwards within it. Slow-growing. Commonest >60y—especially if outdoor occupation
- *Acral lentiginous:* Rare in white-skinned populations; 35%–60% of melanomas in black-skinned patients. Affect palms, soles and nail beds. Often detected late and carries poor prognosis.

Rarer types of melanoma:
- Desmoplastic—contains fibrous scar tissue
- Amelanotic—loses its pigment and appears as a bleached area
- Non-cutaneous—arising in the eye, mouth, under the fingernails, vulval or vaginal tissues, or internally.

Risk factors: Sun exposure is the major risk factor for malignant melanoma. *Other risk factors:*
- Genetic
- Multiple benign moles (>50 of >2mm diameter)
- Congenital nevus
- Previous malignant melanoma
- Immunosuppression
- Fair skin type (red hair, blue eyes and burn easily).

ⓘ 30% malignant melanomas arise out of pre-existing moles but risk of change in a benign mole (except dysplastic or congenital nevus) is small.

Management: Encourage patients to report changes in moles early. Apply the 7-point checklist (📖 p.47) to identify changes needing referral.

Refer: Any suspicious lesions for assessment urgently by a dermatologist ± wide excision. In many areas 'mole clinics' are run for this purpose.

Treatment: Best chance of cure comes with early detection and complete excision. Chemotherapy and radiotherapy are of little benefit except for palliation, but laser therapy and immunotherapy treatment with interferon and/or interleukin-2 are now commonly used. Prognosis relates to tumour depth and spread at presentation (Table 6.18).

Kaposi sarcoma: 📖 p.158

Figure 6.11 Major types of melanoma

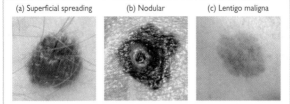

(a) Superficial spreading   (b) Nodular   (c) Lentigo maligna

Figure 6.11 is reproduced with permission from (A) BMJ publishing; (B) Royal College of Surgeons of Edinburgh, and (C) 🖳 www.dermatology.co.uk.

Table 6.18 Thickness of melanoma and survival rates

Breslow thickness	Excision margins (cm)	5y survival (%)
In situ	0.5 or histologically clear	100
<1mm	1	95–100
1–2mm	1–2	80–96
2.1–4mm	2–3 (2 preferred)	60–75
>4mm	2–3	50

ⓘ Patients with palpable/macroscopically involved LNs have <20% 5y survival; patients with disseminated disease have <5% 5y survival.

Reproduced with permission from the British Association of Dermatologists

GP notes

Patients with non-melanotic skin cancer *are not* eligible for inclusion on the practice cancer register. Patients with melanoma *are* eligible for inclusion.

Advice for patients

Further information for patients:

Macmillan Cancer Support ☎ 0808 808 0000
🖳 www.macmillan.org.uk
British Association of Dermatologists 🖳 www.bad.org.uk

149

Further information:

British Association of Dermatologists 🖳 www.bad.org.uk
- Guidelines for the management of BCC (2008)
- Multi-professional guidelines for the management of the patient with primary cutaneous squamous cell carcinoma (2009)
- Guidelines for management of Bowen's disease (2006)
- UK guidelines for the management of cutaneous melanoma (2002)

NICE Improving outcomes for people with skin tumours including melanoma: The Manual (2006) 🖳 www.nice.org.uk

Head and neck tumours

Leukoplakia: Thick whitish, grey patch usually on the inside of the cheek, the tongue or gum. It is the mouth's reaction to chronic irritation of the mucous membranes. ♂ > ♀. Common in patients who smoke, patients with ill-fitting dentures. and patients who habitually chew on their cheek. Usually benign but may be an early sign of oral cancer. NICE recommends referral to oral surgery to exclude malignancy in *all* cases.

Erythroplakia: Reddened area that results when the lining of the mouth thins. The area appears red because the underlying capillaries are more visible. Erythroplakia is a much more ominous predictor of oral cancer than leukoplakia. NICE recommends referral to oral surgery to exclude malignancy in *all* cases

Oral cancer: Usually squamous cell cancer. >5,300 new cases are diagnosed in the UK each year—incidence is increasing. ♂ > ♀. Major risk factors are smoking and high-alcohol consumption. Survival is poor (30%–40% 5y survival) mainly due to poor public awareness and late presentation. Usually presents with:
- Leukoplakia (white patch)
- Erythroplakia (red patch) *or*
- Non-healing ulcer (>3wk).

Management: Refer any suspicious lesions to oral surgery for biopsy. Specialist treatment is with surgery or radiotherapy + chemotherapy.

Malignant melanoma: Malignant melanoma is most common on the hard palate but also occurs on the lower jaw, lips, tongue, or buccal mucosa. It often ulcerates/bleeds. It is infiltrative and metastasizes early to LNs—🔲 p.148.

Carcinoma of the pharynx: Usually SCC, although lymphomas are not unusual, especially if the tonsils or nasopharynx are involved. Lymphomas tend to have better prognosis.

Nasopharyngeal carcinoma: Tumours are often anaplastic and may spread. In the UK, frequently presents with a malignant node in the neck. More common in Asian populations where this tumour is associated with Epstein-Barr virus infection. Other symptoms/signs:
- Nasal obstruction—usually obstruction is bilateral—assume persistent unilateral blockage is neoplastic until proven otherwise
- Nasal polyp—unilateral nasal polyp is tumour until proven otherwise
- Epistaxis
- Otitis media from Eustachian tube obstruction
- Lower cranial nerve palsies from base of skull extension
- IIIrd, IVth, and Vth cranial nerve involvement from cavernous sinus invasion signify advanced disease.

Refer urgently to ENT if suspected. Combined chemoradiotherapy is the treatment of choice. Unusually for head and neck cancers, irradiation of the neck is as effective as radical neck dissection. Xerostomia is common from salivary gland irradiation. Chemotherapy can also be very effective.

GMS contract		
Cancer 1	The practice can produce a register of all cancer patients defined as a 'register' of patients with a diagnosis of cancer excluding non-melanotic skin cancers from 1.4.2003.	5 points
Cancer 3	% of patients with cancer, diagnosed within the last 18mo who have a patient review recorded as occurring within 6mo of the practice receiving confirmation of the diagnosis.	Up to 6 points 40%–90%
Education 7	The practice has undertaken a minimum of 12 significant event reviews in the past 3y which could include (if these have occurred) new cancer diagnoses.	Total of 4 points for 12 significant event reviews

GP notes

🖰 **Malignant transformation of lichen planus:** It is controversial whether oral lichen planus can undergo malignant transformation. If it can, risk is low (<2% over 10y). NICE recommends patients with confirmed oral lichen planus are monitored for oral cancer as part of routine dental examination.

Advice for patients

Support and information for patients:
Mouth Cancer Foundation—information, support and personal experiences of sufferers 🖳 www.rdoc.org.uk
Cancer Research UK (Cancer help UK) ☎ 0808 800 4040
🖳 www.cancerhelp.org.uk
ENT UK 🖳 www.entuk.org

Further information:

SIGN Diganosis and management of head and neck cancer (2006). 🖳 www.sign.ac.uk
NICE Referral guidelines for suspected cancer (2005) 🖳 www.nice.org.uk

Oropharyngeal carcinoma: Affects posterior tongue, soft palate, fauces, tonsils, and/or the pharyngeal wall. Frequently presents late with dysarthria, pain, or aspiration. Refer urgently to ENT if unexplained, persistent sore throat for >1mo or any other suspicious symptoms/signs. Radical chemoradiotherapy is usual but extensive surgery with radical neck dissection followed by radiotherapy may be indicated in locally advanced disease.

Laryngeal carcinoma: There are 2,200 new cases of laryngeal cancer diagnosed each year in the UK and 750 deaths. ♂ > ♀ (4:1). Peak age range is 55–80y. Smoking and alcohol (×2–5) are the main risk factors. These are three types:

- *Glottic (vocal cord)*—most common. Nodal metastases occur late. The first sign is usually hoarseness followed by stridor, dysphagia, and pain
- *Supraglottic*—presents late with vague dysphagia, referred ear pain, and/or cervical LNs. Hoarseness implies involvement of the vocal cords or adjacent structures. Frequently metastasizes to local LNs
- *Subglottic*—rare but highly invasive. Postcricoid tumours may be associated with iron deficiency (Patterson Brown-Kelly syndrome).

Management: Refer any patient with hoarseness persisting >3wk for urgent CXR. If CXR is negative or any other symptoms/signs suggesting laryngeal carcinoma, refer urgently to ENT. Diagnosis is confirmed with laryngoscopy and biopsy. Treatment is with surgery ± radiotherapy. Overall survival is ~60%. Early tumours confined to the vocal cord have 80—90% 5y survival. Chemoradiotherapy in advanced cases is associated with laryngeal preservation.

Salivary gland tumours: 80% of tumours are in the parotid gland. Usually present with a swelling or lump in a salivary gland. Types:

- *Adenoid cystic carcinoma:* Most common salivary cancer. It is slow growing and ulcerative. It is the tumour most likely to spread along perineural sheaths, leading to nerve palsies and neuropathic pain. It also infiltrates marrow cavities, so X-ray may miss its true extent
- *Adenocarcinoma*
- *SCC:* More aggressive than adenocarcinoma—cause pain, and metastasize early. More often metastatic than primary
- *Undifferentiated carcinoma:* Progresses rapidly. May mimic sarcoma
- A very small proportion of *pleomorphic adenomas* become malignant.

Referral: Refer urgently to ENT/oral surgery if >1mo, unexplained swelling in the parotid or submandibular gland. Refer earlier if signs of malignancy:

- Pain
- Rapid growth
- Hard fixed mass
- Weight ↓
- Facial nerve palsy.

Treatment and prognosis: Specialist management is with surgery. Radiotherapy is used for residual or recurrent disease, high-grade tumours, or lymphomas. The facial nerve may be involved by tumour or sacrificed at operation

Carcinoma of the thyroid: Uncommon cancer causing 2,000 new cases of cancer/y in the UK. ♀ > ♂ (3:1)—most common in South Asian women. Risk goes up with age in men until 75y; in women risk peaks aged 30–55y and then ↓. Risk factors include benign thyroid disease; past history of neck irradiation; family history of thyroid cancer, multiple endocrine neoplasia or familial adenomatous polyposis; low-iodine levels; poor diet (high intake of butter, cheese and meat may cause 40% of cases).

Presentation:
- Solid thyroid nodule increasing in size
- Unexplained hoarseness or voice changes
- Cervical lymphadenopathy
- Stridor/breathlessness due to thyroid swelling—immediate referral/admission.

Primary tumours:
- *Papillary adenocarcinoma* (60%): Typical age range: 10–40y. ♀ > ♂. Low-grade malignancy which is rarely fatal. Spread occurs to local LNs and/or lung. The tumour is sensitive to thyroid stimulating hormone so following thyroidectomy treatment with thyroxine continues lifelong
- *Follicular carcinoma* (25%): Typical age range: 40–60y. ♀ > ♂. May arise in a pre-existing multinodular goitre. Metastasizes via the bloodstream and boney secondaries are common. Treatment is with surgery and thyroxine suppression therapy and/or radioactive iodine
- *Anaplastic carcinoma* (rare): Typical age range: 50–60y. ♀ > ♂. Aggressive tumour that grows rapidly and infiltrates the tissues of the neck. Compression of the trachea is common. Metastasizes locally to LNs and via lymphatics. Poor response to treatment
- *Medullary carcinoma* (rare): Occurs at any age. ♀ = ♂. Familial incidence; associated with adenomas elsewhere. Often secretes calcitonin which is used as a tumour marker. Spreads to local LNs. Treated by excision then chemotherapy ± radiotherapy
- *Lymphoma* (5%): Occurs at any age. May be primary or secondary. May be associated with Hashimoto's thyroiditis. Staged and treated as for lymphomas elsewhere (📖 p.140). Prognosis is good.

Advice for patients

Information for patients:
Cancer Research UK (Cancer help UK) ☎ 0808 800 4040
🖥 www.cancerhelp.org.uk
ENT UK 🖥 www.entuk.org
British Thyroid Foundation 🖥 www.btf-thyroid.org

Other cancers

Sarcoma: is cancer of the bone or connective tissue. In total 1,850 patients are diagnosed each year in the UK with sarcoma and it causes 1,000 deaths. There are two peaks of incidence—one in teenagers and another in old age. Five types of sarcoma account for >80% of tumours:

Osteosarcoma and the Ewing's family of tumours: Present with aching bone pain, swelling ± pathological fracture. Refer for X-ray if:
- Fracture is suspected or
- Increasing, unexplained, or persistent bone pain or tenderness, particularly pain at rest (and especially if not in the joint), or
- Unexplained limp.

⊕ In older people consider metastases, myeloma or lymphoma, as well as sarcoma.

Management: Refer to orthopaedics as an emergency or urgently, depending on circumstances, if fracture on X-ray or X-ray shows bone cancer. If X-ray is normal but symptoms persist, consider checking bone function tests, re-X-raying, discussing the patient with a specialist, or consider referral. Treatment involves surgery and chemotherapy. Overall 5y survival is 50%–80%.

Adult soft tissue sarcomas of limb, limb girdle, and trunk: Refer urgently if a patient presents with a palpable lump that is:
- >5cm in diameter
- Increasing in size
- Deep to fascia, fixed, or immobile
- Painful
- A recurrence after previous excision.

⊕ If a patient has HIV consider Kaposi sarcoma.

The most common tumours are leiomyosarcoma, liposarcoma, and synovial sarcoma. Surgery is the mainstay of treatment although high-grade tumours are usually also treated with radiotherapy. Chemotherapy is of modest benefit for many sarcomas and is usually reserved for palliation

Kaposi's sarcoma: May be associated with immunosuppression, when tends to be more aggressive. This condition presents with nodules in the skin (Figure 6.12), mucus membranes, GI tract, or lungs and spreads to LNs and/or liver, especially in immunocompromised patients. Lymphatic obstruction predisposes to cellulitis. If suspected refer urgently for specialist opinion. Treatment varies according to site and dissemination and can be topical (cryotherapy, topical chemotherapy), surgical (excision), or involve radiotherapy, and/or systemic chemotherapy. If Kaposi sarcoma is a presenting feature of HIV infection, treatment with highly active anti-retroviral therapy (HAART) alone may induce remission.

Intra-abdominal sarcomas: Usually present late. Often arise in the retroperitoneum. If possible, surgery is the main treatment. Local relapse is common and often not responsive to cytotoxic therapy.

Rhabdomyosarcoma: This originates from striated muscle and presents usually in children <2y with a lump. Responds to intensive multi-modal therapy; outlook is generally good with >60% long-term survival.

Figure 6.12 Kaposi sarcoma on a hand

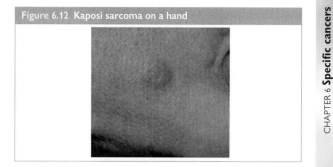

GMS contract

Cancer 1	The practice can produce a register of all cancer patients defined as a 'register' of patients with a diagnosis of cancer excluding non-melanotic skin cancers from 1.4.2003.	5 points	
Cancer 3	% of patients with cancer, diagnosed within the last 18mo who have a patient review recorded as occurring within 6mo of the practice receiving confirmation of the diagnosis.	Up to 6 points	40%–90%
Education 7	The practice has undertaken a minimum of 12 significant event reviews in the past 3y which could include (if these have occurred) new cancer diagnoses.	Total of 4 points for 12 significant event reviews	

Advice for patients

Information and support for patients:
Sarcoma UK ⌨ www.sarcoma-uk.org
Macmillan Cancer Support ☎ 0808 808 0000
⌨ www.macmillan.org.uk
Cancer Research UK ☎ 0808 800 4040 ⌨ www.cancerhelp.org.uk

Phaechromocytoma: Rare but serious disorder affecting 0.1% hypertensive patients. Peak age 30–40y. Usually caused by catecholamine secreting tumours—10% are bilateral (70% if familial), 10% extra-adrenal (usually aortic bifurcation); 10% occur in children; 10% are malignant.

Presentation: May present with a huge array of symptoms and signs. ↑ BP may be sporadic or sustained. Suspect in:
- Young patients with ↑ BP
- Patients with high BP which responds poorly to anti-hypertensives
- Patients with very labile BP *or*
- If associated headaches, sweating and/or palpitations.

Other symptoms include the following: headache, palpitations/tachycardia, sweating, tremor/anxiety/panic attacks; nausea and vomiting; fever.

🅘 May be associated with other conditions (e.g. neurofibromatosis—5%; multiple endocrine neoplasia; von Hippel-Lindau syndrome). Every patient with a phaeochromocytoma should be screened for von Hippel-Lindau and multiple endocrine neoplasia (MEN-II).

Differential diagnosis: Includes the following:
- Essential hypertension, pre-eclampsia, eclampsia, or simple hypertension of pregnancy
- Thyrotoxicosis
- Migraine
- Alcohol withdrawal
- Carcinoid syndrome
- Hypoglycaemia
- Angina pectoris.

Investigation: 24h urine collection ×3 for urinary free catecholamines (adrenaline and noradrenaline), or their metabolites e.g. vanillylmandelic acid (VMA) or 4-hydroxy-3-methoxymandelic acid (HMMA). 2× normal levels are diagnostic. Avoid ingestion of coffee, bananas, and vanilla flavouring for 24h before collection.

Management: Refer for specialist opinion if suspected. Treatment is usually surgical and curative in 75%.

Multiple endocrine neoplasia (MEN): Autosomal dominant inherited predisposition to tumours of endocrine glands. Often, only one major lesion is evident clinically but other asymptomatic tumours are present and discovered when investigated directly. There are two types:

MEN I: 20 cases/y in the UK. Patients are prone to tumours of the:
- *Parathyroid gland*—>90%. Result in hypercalcaemia ± hyperparathyroidism
- *Pancreatic islets*—usually multiple tumours (75%). Include gastrinoma (most common—can lead to Zollinger–Ellison syndrome), insulinoma, VIPoma, or glucagonoma
- *Anterior pituitary gland*—50%—Most secrete prolactin, growth hormone, or ACTH
- *Carcinoid*—less common
- *Adrenal cortex*—less common.

MEN-II: There are two variants:

MEN-IIA: 95% cases. Patients have:
- Medullary carcinoma of the thyroid—>90%—usually very slow growing
- Multiple phaeochromocytomas in the adrenal medulla—50%—major cause of death
- Parathyroid hyperplasia or adenoma—less common.

MEN-IIB (or MEN-III): 5% cases.
- Medullary carcinoma of the thyroid
- Phaeochromocytoma
- Mucosal neuromas of lips, eyelids, and tongue
- Neuromas of the ganglions of the bowel
- Marfanoid habitus (spider fingers, long arms/legs, high-arched palate)
- Proximal myopathy.

🕕 Up to a quarter of patients with phaeochromocytoma will have MEN-II or von Hippel-Lindau syndrome rare autosomal dominant disorder in which haemangioblastomas are found in the retina, spinal canal, and cerebellum). Every patient with a phaeochromocytoma should be screened for both.

Unknown primary: Some patients present with metastatic disease. Despite all our advances in imaging and endoscopy, carcinoma of unknown primary represents approximately 5% of all malignant disease. Although the cell type, or tumour markers, may give clues to the organ of origin, sometimes the primary tumour cannot be found. This can occur for two reasons—the primary tumour may be too small to detect or the primary tumour may no longer be present (e.g. destroyed by the patient's immune system). Depending on the age and state of the patient, location of secondary tumour, cell types or tumour markers found, treatment with chemotherapy (and sometimes radiotherapy) may be offered.

Childhood cancer

Every year in the UK, 1,500 children are diagnosed with cancer and 300 children die as a result of cancer. The most common type of cancer in childhood is acute leukaemia (1:3) followed by brain tumour (1:4). Risk of developing cancer for an individual child is 71:500 and 75% developing cancer will survive 5y. Following treatment, if a child survives 5y there is only a 10% chance of death from tumour recurrence or treatment effects.

Acute leukaemia: 📖 p.132

Lymphoma: 📖 p.136

Brain tumours: 📖 p.144

Sarcoma: 📖 p.154

Neuroblastoma: Tumour derived from neural crest tissue. 80 cases/y are reported in England and Wales—8% of all paediatric tumours. Neuroblastoma tends to affect children <4y old (50% <2y; 90%<9y). *Sites:* adrenal medulla—50%; abdominal sympathetic ganglia—25%; chest—20%; pelvis—5%; neck—5%.

Presentation: Variable and often non-specific—depends on site of the tumour and extent of metastases. ~half present with metastatic disease.
- *General effects:*
  - Pallor
  - Fever
  - Anorexia and weight ↓
  - Irritability
  - Flushing
  - Ataxia
  - Diarrhoea
  - Failure to thrive.
- *Local effects of the tumour:* Abdominal mass (or thoracic mass on CXR); local spread may cause paraplegia or cauda equine syndrome. Infants <6mo may have rapidly progressive intra-abdominal disease
- *Effects of metastases:* Lymphatic and haematogenous spread, particularly to liver, lungs, and bone, is common. Associated symptoms:
  - Bone pain ± pathological fracture
  - Breathlessness
  - Periorbital bruising (looks like a black eye), proptosis or Horner syndrome
  - Firm skin nodules (usually babies—'blueberry muffin appearance').

Investigate with a FBC if: Persistent or unexplained bone pain (X-ray is also needed); pallor or fatigue; unexplained irritability; unexplained fever; persistent or recurrent UTI; generalized lymphadenopathy; and/or unexplained bruising.

If neuroblastoma is suspected: Carry out an abdominal examination (and/or urgent USS), and consider CXR and FBC. If any mass is found, refer urgently.

Specialist management and prognosis: Treatment is with surgery, chemotherapy, and/or radiotherapy. Early stage disease has a 95% 5y survival; late-stage disease has 20% 5y survival. Children with extra-abdominal tumours and those who are <1y at diagnosis have better prognosis.

Wilm's nephroblastoma: 70 cases/y in England and Wales. Kidney tumour composed of primitive renal tissue. The left kidney is affected more often than the right and it is bilateral in 10%. It usually affects children <5y old (peak age: 2–3y). ♂ > ♀. Rarely associated with Beckwith-Wiedemann syndrome, aniridia, or hemihypertrophy.

Presentation:
- *General effects:* Fever, anorexia, and weight ↓, anaemia
- *Local effects of the tumour:* Unilateral abdominal mass ± pain ± unexplained haematuria
- *Effects of metastases:* 20% have metastases to liver, lungs, or bone (rare) at presentation. May present with symptoms/signs of metastases.

Management: If a child presents with abdominal distension, examine the abdomen. *Refer if:* Intra-abdominal mass (immediate referral) or unexplained haematuria (urgent referral).

Specialist treatment and prognosis: Treatment is with surgery ± chemotherapy ± radiotherapy depending on histology and stage at diagnosis. Early stage tumours have 80% 5y survival; late-stage tumours have 50% 5y survival.

Retinoblastoma: Rare tumour of the eye. Approximately 30 cases/y occur in England and Wales. This usually affects children <1y old— most are <5y old. May be familial (6%—dominant inheritance) when the tumour is usually bilateral. Sporadic tumours are usually unilateral.

Presentation:
- Usually detected by a white papillary reflex found at routine developmental screening (Figure 3.1, 📖 p.51)
- Alternatively may present with squint or inflammation of the eye.

Management: Refer suspected cases for urgent ophthalmology opinion.

Specialist treatment and prognosis: Treatment of unilateral tumours is surgical. Bilateral tumours are treated by enucleation or laser ablation of the worst affected eye and radiotherapy to the other eye. Approximately 80% patients with unilateral tumours survive long term. Bilateral tumours have a poorer prognosis with 40% surviving long term.

Further information:
NICE Referral guidelines for suspected cancer (2005) 🖥 www.nice.org.uk

159

Advice for patients

Information and support for patients and their carers:
Neuroblastoma society ☎ 020 8940 4353 🖥 www.nsoc.co.uk
Childhood eye cancer trust (CHECT) ☎ 020 7377 5578
🖥 www.chect.org.uk

Chapter 7

Palliative care

Palliative care in general practice

'Any man's death diminishes me because I am involved in mankind'
Devotions Meditation 17, John Donne 1572–1631.

Palliative care starts when the emphasis changes from curing the patient and prolonging life to relieving symptoms and maintaining well-being or 'quality of life'. GPs have 1–2 patients with terminal disease at any time and get more personally involved with them than any others.

The problems arising are a complex mix of physical, psychological, social, cultural, and spiritual factors involving both patients and carers. To respond adequately good lines of communication and close multi-disciplinary teamwork is needed. Local palliative care teams are invaluable sources of advice and support and frequently produce booklets with advice on aspects of palliative care for GPs.

Weakness, fatigue, and drowsiness: These are almost universal symptoms.

Reversible causes:
- Drugs—opioids, benzodiazepines, steroids (proximal muscle weakness), diuretics (dehydration and biochemical abnormalities), anti-hypertensives (postural hypotension)
- Emotional problems—depression, anxiety, fear, apathy
- Hypercalcaemia
- Other biochemical abnormalities—DM, electrolyte disturbance, uraemia, liver disease, thyroid dysfunction
- Anaemia
- Poor nutrition
- Infection
- Prolonged bed rest
- Raised intra-cranial pressure (drowsiness only).

Management:
- Treat reversible causes
- If drowsiness and fatigue persist consider a trial of dexamethasone 4–6 mg/d. or anti-depressant. Although steroids make muscle wasting worse they may improve general fatigue and improve mobility
- Psychological support of patients and carers—empathy, explanation
- Physical support—referral to physiotherapist, review of aids and appliances, review of home layout (possibly with referral to occupational therapy), review of home care arrangements
- Advice on modification of lifestyle.

162

Further information:
Gold Standards Framework ☎ 01922 604666
🖥 www.goldstandardsframework.nhs.uk
NICE Improving supportive and palliative care for adults with cancer (2004) 🖥 www.nice.org.uk
Hospice information ☎ 020 7520 8222 🖥 www.hospiceinformation.info
Oxford GP library *Pain and palliation* (2010) OUP ISBN: 9780199215720
Watson et al. *Oxford Handbook of Palliative Care* (2005) Oxford University Press ISBN: 0198508972
Woodruff and Doyle *The IAHPC Manual of Palliative Care* (2nd Edition) IAHPC Press (2004) ISBN 0-9758525-1-5
🖥 www.hospicecare.com/manual/IAHPCmanual.htm

GP Notes

Basic rules of symptom control: Symptom control must be tailored to the needs of the individual.

- Carefully diagnose the cause of the symptom
- Explain the symptom to the patient
- Discuss treatment options
- Set realistic goals
- Anticipate likely problems
- Review regularly.

⚠ Death is the natural end to life—not a failure of medicine.

Advice for patients

Advice and support for patients:
Macmillan Cancer Support ☎ 0808 808 0000
🖫 www.macmillan.org.uk

GMS contract

Palliative care 3	The practice has a complete register of all patients in need of palliative care/support regardless of age.	3 points
Palliative care 2	The practice has multi-disciplinary case review meetings at least every 3mo where all patients on the palliative care register are discussed.	3 points

Pain control

Pain control is the cornerstone of palliative care. Three quarters of cancer patients have some pain. Cancer pain is multifactorial—be aware of physical and psychological factors. The majority of pain can be managed using a step-by-step approach to pain relief (Figure 7.1).

Step 1: Non-opioid:

- Start with paracetamol 1g every 4–6h regularly (maximum dose 4g/d)
- If this is not adequate in 24h, stop and either try an NSAID e.g. ibuprofen 400mg tds (if appropriate) alone or in combination with paracetamol, or proceed to step 2.

Step 2: Weak opioid + non-opioid:

- Start treatment with a combined preparation of paracetamol with codeine or dihydrocodeine. Combining two analgesics with different mechanisms of action enables better pain control than using either drug alone at that dose
- Combinations have ↓ dose-related side effects but the range of side effects is ↑ (additive effects of two drugs). Combinations using full-dose opioid (e.g. Solpadol®) are more effective than paracetamol alone but it is cheaper and more flexible to prescribe constituents separately e.g. 'paracetamol 500mg/codeine 30mg'
- Advise patients to take tablets regularly and not to assess efficacy after only a couple of doses.

 There is no additional analgesic benefit from preparations which contain paracetamol + 8mg of codeine, as opposed to paracetamol alone.

Step 3: Strong opioid + non-opioid:

- Use immediate-release morphine tablets or morphine solution depending on patient preference. Two tablets of co-codamol contain 60mg of codeine which is equi-analgesic to ~6mg of oral morphine. If changing to morphine, use a minimum dose of 5mg
- Chronic pain may not respond to opioids. Give for a 2wk trial and only continue if of proven benefit. Worries of tolerance/addiction are unfounded for patients with true opioid-sensitive pain. If the pain seems responsive to opioids and there are no undue side effects, ↑ the dose upwards by 30%–50% every 24h until pain is controlled—📖 p.172.

⚠ If the patient is elderly or in renal failure—consider starting with a ↓ dose of morphine.

Addition of co-analgesics and adjuvant drugs: These drugs in combination with analgesics can enhance pain control. Examples include:

- *Antidepressants*—for nerve pain and depression associated with pain
- *Anticonvulsants*—e.g. gabapentin for neuropathic pain
- *Corticosteroids*—pain due to oedema
- *Muscle relaxants*—muscle cramp pain
- *Antispasmodics*—bowel colic
- *Antibiotics*—pain associated with infection
- *Night sedative*—when lack of sleep is lowering pain threshold
- *Anxiolytic*—if anxiety makes pain worse (relaxation may also help).

Figure 7.1 World Health Organization analgesics ladder

		Step 3
	Step 2	**Severe pain** Strong opioids e.g. morphine, hydro- morphone, diamorphine, buprenorphine, fentanyl transdermal therapeutic system (TTS) patch
Step 1	**Moderate pain** Weak opioids e.g. tramadol, dihydrocodeine	
Mild pain Non-opioids e.g. NSAID and/or paracetamol	± non-opioid (paracetamol and/or NSAID)	± non-opioid (paracetamol and/or NSAID)

Co-analgesics: drugs, nerve blocks, TENS, relaxation, acupuncture

Specific therapies: surgery, physiotherapy

Address psychosocial problems

GP notes

Trouble shooting:

- Continuing pain and frequent prn doses -↑ regular dose
- Persisting side effects (drowsiness, jerking, vomiting, confusion)—↓ regular dose
- Considerable pain despite marked side effects—use alternative.

Quick conversions:

From	To	Conversion	Example
Oral *morphine* *(total dose)* *e.g. 10mg* *morphine* *four hourly* *= 60mg oral* *morphine in* *24h.*	SC diamorphine	÷ by 3	60 ÷ 3 = 20mg diamorphine by syringe driver over 24h.
	SC morphine	÷ by 2	60 ÷ 2 = 30mg morphine by syringe driver over 24h.
	oral oxycodone	÷ by 2	60 ÷ 2 = 30mg oral oxycodone in divided doses over 24h.
	oral hydro- morphone	÷ by 7.5	60 ÷ 7.5 = (60 × 2) ÷ 15 = 8mg hydromorphone in divided doses over 24h.

ⓘ If total 24h dose is equivalent to 360mg morphine or more—get specialist advice.

Opioid toxicity: May be increased by dehydration, renal failure, other analgesics (e.g. NSAIDs), and co-administration of amitriptyline. Symptoms:

- Drowsiness, coma, or confusion—including auditory/visual hallucinations
- Vomiting
- Respiratory depression—📖 p.95
- Pinpoint pupils
- Hypotension
- Muscle rigidity/myoclonus—consider renal failure (can produce myoclonus alone). Treat by rehydration, stopping other medication which may exacerbate myoclonus, switching opioid or with clonazepam 2–4mg/24h depending on circumstances.

Table 7.1 Management of specific types of pain

Type of pain	Management
Bone pain	• Try NSAIDs and/or strong opioids • Consider referral for palliative radiotherapy, strontium treatment (prostate cancer), or IV bisphosphonates (↓ pain in myeloma, breast, and prostate cancer) • Refer to orthopaedics if any lytic metastases at risk of fracture, for consideration of pinning.
Abdominal pain	• Constipation is the most common cause—📖 p.176 • Colic—try loperamide 2–4mg qds or hyoscine hydrobromide 300mcg tds sublingual. Hyoscine butylbromide (Buscopan®) 20–60mg/24h can also be given via syringe driver • Liver capsule pain—dexamethasone 4–8mg/d. Titrate dose ↓ to the minimum that controls pain. Alternatively try an NSAID + proton pump inhibitor cover • Gastric distention—may be helped by an antacid, ± an anti-foaming agent (e.g. Asilone®). Alternatively a prokinetic may help e.g. domperidone 10mg tds before meals • Upper GI tumour—often neuropathic element of pain—coeliac plexus block may help—refer to palliative care • Consider drug causes—NSAIDs are a common cause • Acute/subacute obstruction—📖 p.175.
Neuropathic pain	• Often burning/shooting and may not respond to simple analgesia • Titrate to the maximum tolerated dose of opioid • If inadequate add a nerve pain killer e.g. amitriptyline 10–25mg nocte increasing as needed every 2wk to 75–150mg. Alternatives include carbamazepine, gabapentin, pregabalin, phenytoin, sodium valproate, and clonazepam • If pain is due to nerve compression due to tumour, dexamethasone 4–8 mg od may help • *Other options:* TENS; acupuncture; nerve block; radiotherapy.
Rectal pain	• Topical drugs e.g. rectal steroids • Tricyclic antidepressants e.g. amitriptyline 10–100mg nocte • Anal spasms—glyceryl trinitrate ointment 0.1%–0.2% bd • Referral for local radiotherapy.
Muscle pain	• Paracetamol and/or NSAIDs • Muscle relaxants e.g. diazepam 5–10mg od, baclofen 5–10mg tds, dantrolene 25mg od increasing at weekly intervals to 75mg tds • Physiotherapy, aromatherapy, relaxation, heat pads.
Bladder pain/ spasm	• Treat reversible causes. ↑ fluids. Toilet regularly • Try oxybutynin 5mg tds, tolterodine 2mg bd, propiverine 15mg od/bd/tds, or trospium 20mg bd • Amitriptyline 10–75mg nocte is often effective. NSAIDs can also be useful (if not contraindicated) • If catheterized—try instilling 20ml of intravesical bupivacaine 0.25% for 15min tds • Steroids e.g. dexamethasone—4–8mg od may ↓ tumour-related bladder inflammation. • In the terminal situation hyoscine butylbromide 60–120mg/24h or glycopyrronium 0.4–0.8mg/24h SCcan be helpful.
Pain of short duration	• E.g. dressing changes—try a short-acting opioid e.g. Fentanyl citrate 200mcg lozenge sucked for 15min before the procedure or a breakthrough dose of oral morphine 20min before the procedure.

Starting a patient on morphine: If possible start with immediate-release morphine liquid or tablets depending on the patient preference. Four hourly morphine gives greatest flexibility for initial dose titration and causes fewer side effects than longer-acting preparations. If less severe pain or difficulties with compliance, consider starting with a bd modified release (m/r) preparation. Give clear instructions.

Initial dosage:
- *Adults not pain-controlled with regular weak opioids* (e.g. co-codamol 500/30 two tablets qds)—5mg oral morphine every 4h (or 15mg m/r morphine every 12h)
- *Elderly, cachectic, or not taking regular weak opioids*—2.5mg–5mg of morphine every 4h (or 15–20mg of m/r morphine every 12h)
- *Very elderly and frail*—2.5mg of morphine every 4h (or 15mg of m/r morphine every 12h).

Prevention of adverse effects:
- Always prescribe a laxative concurrently (e.g. docusate, bisacodyl)
- >1:3 patients develop nausea on starting opioids—prescribe a regular antiemetic e.g. haloperidol 1.5mg nocte. Opioid-induced nausea wears off in <2wk, so antiemetics can be stopped after 2wk
- Explain any drowsiness will usually wear off after a few days. Advise patients not to drive for at least 1wk. after starting morphine or after any increase in dose. Patients should also avoid driving after this time if drowsiness persists.

Breakthrough pain: This is pain of rapid onset, moderate/severe intensity, and short duration which may be precipitated by activity but can occur spontaneously. *Management:*
- Ensure access to immediate-release morphine for breakthrough pain. Give the same dose as the four hourly dose as an additional dose
- If pain starts to occur regularly before the next dose of analgesia is due, increase the regular *background dose.*

Titration of dose: Increase the dose as needed by increments of 25%–50% daily until pain is controlled or side effects prevent further increase. There is no 'maximum' daily allowance. e.g. 5→10→15→20→30→40→60→80→100→130→160→200mg

ⓘ Very few patients require more than 600mg daily.

Maintenance: Once pain is controlled, if the patient is taking four hourly doses of morphine, consider switching to a long-acting preparation of equivalent dosage (e.g. MST® bd or MXL® od). Calculate total daily dose of morphine by adding together the four hourly doses. This is the od dosage. The bd dosage can be obtained by dividing the total dosage by two.

Further information:

SIGN Management of pain in adults with cancer (2008)
🖥 www.sign.ac.uk

Drugs and Therapeutics Bulletin Opioid analgesics for cancer pain in primary care (2005)

Mouth problems

Mouth problems affect up to 60% of patients with advanced cancer and can impact greatly on quality of life—both physically and psychologically. The majority of mouth problems seen in palliative care are related to a ↓ in saliva secretion and/or poor oral hygiene.

Risk factors:
- ↓ oral intake
- Debility and ↓ ability to perform self-care
- Dry mouth—due to dehydration, medication, radiotherapy, anxiety, mouth breathing, oxygen therapy
- Weight loss—results in poor fitting dentures
- Anaemia—iron deficiency anaemia causes angular stomatitis/glossitis
- Vitamin C deficiency—causes gingivitis and bleeding gums
- Treatment side effects—local irradiation or chemotherapy
- Local tumour.

Assessment: Assess regularly for symptoms/signs of mouth problems e.g. altered taste, pain and/or mouth ulcers, dry mouth, halitosis, thrush, or dental problems. Consider checking FBC for iron deficiency anaemia.

General measures:
- Keep mouth moist—encourage regular sips of fluids and/or rinsing
- Clean teeth/dentures regularly—if the patient is unable to do it for him/herself instruct carers on mouth care
- Gently clean the tongue with a soft toothbrush or sponge
- Apply moisturizing cream or petroleum jelly (Vaseline®) to lips
- Review medication making the mouth sore or dry
- Mouthwashes—saline 0.9% mouthwashes help removal of oral debris and are soothing
- Consider referral to the district nurse or palliative care home nursing team for advice
- Consider referral to the dentist, ear, nose and throat, or palliative care if symptoms are not settling.

Specific measures: See Table 7.2.

Oral thrush (candidiasis): Infection presents with sore mouth ± loss of taste ± dysphagia. Examination reveals white plaques visible on the buccal mucosa which can be wiped off ± angular stomatitis.

Management:
- Remove tongue deposits with a toothbrush by brushing 2×/d.
- Treat with oral pastilles, suspensions, or gels (e.g. nystatin suspension 100,000 U/ml 2–5ml qds po for 1–2wk)
- If false teeth advise to place imidazole gel on the teeth before insertion and sterilize by soaking for >12h (usually overnight) with dilute hypochlorite solution (e.g. Milton) to prevent re-infection
- Reserve systemic treatment (e.g. oral fluconazole 50mg od for 1–2wk) for patients with recurrent, extensive, systemic, or resistant infection
- Higher doses/prolonged therapy may be needed if immunosuppressed—seek specialist advice.

Table 7.2 Specific measures for treatment of mouth problems

Problem	Treatment options
Dry mouth	Review medication which might be causing dryness e.g. opioids, anti-depressants.
	Hydrate as well as possible.
	Consider salivary stimulants (especially before-meals)—iced water/sucking ice cubes, pineapple chunks, chewing gum, boiled sweets or mints.
	Consider saliva substitutes e.g. Glandosane® spray, Oralbalance® gel.
	Radiotherapy-induced dryness—consider pilocarpine 5mg po tds (sweating is a common side effect), pilocarpine 4% eye drops in raspberry syrup or peppermint water 2–3 drops po tds (unlicensed) or Bethanechol 10mg tds with meals.
Mouth ulcers/sore patches	Topical analgesia e.g. Teejel®, Bonjela®.
	Hydrocortisone lozenges (Corlan®) 1 qds po to ulcerated area.
	Tetracycline mouthwash—for resistant ulcers—dissolve contents of a 250mg capsule in water and hold in the mouth for 2–3min bd for 3d. Avoid swallowing. May stain teeth.
	Chemotherapy-induced ulcers—sucralfate suspension 10ml as mouthwash every 4h.
Cancer pain	Try topical NSAIDs e.g. ibuprofen dispersible 200–400mg tds
Excessive salivation/drooling	Non-drug treatment—head positioning, suction.
	Amitriptyline 10–100mg po.
	Propantheline 15mg tds.
	β-blockers e.g. atenolol 50mg od.
	Atropine eye drops two drops to mouth qds (unlicensed).
Generally sore mouth	Avoid foods that trigger pain e.g. acidic foods.
	Consider systemic analgesic e.g. NSAID and/or opioids.
	Difflam® mouthwash 10ml qds (dilute in same amount of water before use if stings).
	Soluble aspirin—rinse mouth and swallow—300–600mg qds if no contraindications.
	Lidocaine spray, gel, or cream—beware of pharyngeal anaesthesia and risk of aspiration.
	Povidone iodine (Betadine®), hexetidine (Oraldene®), or chlorhexidine 0.2% (Corsodyl®) mouthwash—rinse with 10ml for 1 min bd.
Oral infection	Thrush—see opposite page.
	Cold sores (HSV infection)—if presents early, treat with topical aciclovir 5×/d. If immunocompromised, severe infection, or systemic infection, admit for IV aciclovir.
Coated tongue/mouth	Use a soft toothbrush/sponge to clean the tongue.
	A quarter–half an ascorbic acid 1g effervescent tablet/d. can help—place on tongue and allow to dissolve.
	Fresh pineapple contains enzymes which dissolve the protein coating—try sucking small pieces.

169

Cough and breathlessness

Cough: Cough is a troublesome symptom. Prolonged bouts of coughing are exhausting and frightening—especially if associated with breathlessness and/or haemoptysis.

Breathlessness: Affects 70% of terminally ill patients. It is usually multifactorial. Breathlessness always has a psychological element—being short of breath is frightening. Causes—Figure 7.2.

Management:
General non-drug measures:
- Generally reassure. Explain reasons for breathlessness/cough and adaptations to lifestyle that might help e.g. sitting up straight
- Breathing exercises can help—refer to physiotherapy
- Exclude treatable causes (Box 7.1 and Figure 7.2)
- Steam inhalations or nebulized saline can help with tenacious secretions
- Try a stream of air over the face if the patient is breathless e.g. fan, open window.

General drug measures:
- Try simple linctus 5–10ml prn for cough
- Oral or subcutaneous opioids ↓ subjective sensation of breathlessness—start with 2.5mg oral morphine four hourly and titrate upwards. Opioids may also help with cough—try pholcodeine 10ml tds or oral morphine as for breathlessness. If already on opioids, ↑ dose by 25%. Titrate dose until symptoms are controlled or side effects
- Try benzodiazepines—2–5mg diazepam od/bd for background control of breathlessness + lorazepam 1–2mg sublingual prn in between. Diazepam acts as a central cough suppressant—try 2–10mg tds for cough
- Oxygen has a variable effect and is worth a try
- Hyoscine 400–600 mcg 4–8hourly (or 0.6–2.4mg/24h via syringe driver) and/or ipratropium inhalers/nebulized ipratropium ↓ secretions.

Specific measures:
- *Chest infection*—treat with nebulized saline to make secretions less viscous ±antibiotics (if not considered a terminal event)
- *Post-nasal drip*—steam inhalations, steroid nasal spray, or drops ± antibiotics
- *Laryngeal irritation*—try inhaled steroids e.g. beclometasone 100mcg/actuation two puffs bd
- *Bronchospasm*—try bronchodilators ± inhaled or oral steroids
  ! salbutamol may help cough even in the absence of wheeze.
- *Gastric reflux*—try antacids containing dimethicone (Gaviscon®, Asilone®)
- *Lung cancer*—try inhaled sodium cromoglicate 10mg qds; local anaesthesia using nebulized bupivacaine or lidocaine can be helpful—refer for specialist advice (avoid eating/drinking for 1h afterwards to avoid aspiration). Palliative radiotherapy or chemotherapy can also relieve cough in patients with lung cancer—refer.

Haemoptysis: 📖 p.84   **Pulmonary embolus**: 📖 p.87

Superior vena cava obstruction: 📖 p.87

Figure 7.2 Causes of breathlessness

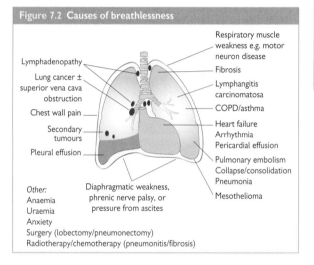

Lymphadenopathy

Lung cancer ± superior vena cava obstruction

Chest wall pain

Secondary tumours

Pleural effusion

Respiratory muscle weakness e.g. motor neuron disease

Fibrosis

Lymphangitis carcinomatosa

COPD/asthma

Heart failure
Arrhythmia
Pericardial effusion

Pulmonary embolism
Collapse/consolidation
Pneumonia

Mesothelioma

Diaphragmatic weakness, phrenic nerve palsy, or pressure from ascites

Other:
Anaemia
Uraemia
Anxiety
Surgery (lobectomy/pneumonectomy)
Radiotherapy/chemotherapy (pneumonitis/fibrosis)

GP tip

Anaemia: Don't check for anaemia if there is no intention to transfuse.
- *If Hb <10g/dl and symptomatic:* treat any reversible cause (e.g. iron deficiency, GI bleeding secondary to NSAIDs). Consider transfusion
- *If transfused:* record whether any benefit is derived (as if not, further transfusions are futile) and the duration of benefit (if <3wk— repeat transfusions are impractical). Monitor for return of symptoms, repeat FBC and arrange repeat transfusion as needed.

Further information:

Doyle *et al.* *Oxford Textbook of Palliative Medicine* (2005) OUP ISBN: 0198566980

Nausea and vomiting

Nausea and vomiting are common symptoms which cause patients and their relative's deep distress. Of the two, nausea causes most misery.

General principles of management:
- *Assess*—try to identify likely cause—Table 7.3
- *Review medication*—could medication be the cause? Which anti-emetics have been used before and how effective were they?
- *Try non-drug measures* (see below)
- *Choose an antiemetic*—if cause can be identified, choose an antiemetic appropriate for the cause (Table 7.3). Use the antiemetic ladder (Figure 7.3). Administer antiemetics regularly rather than prn and choose an appropriate route of administration (see below)
- *Review frequently*—is the antiemetic effective? Has the underlying cause of the nausea/vomiting resolved? Avoid changing antiemetic before it has been given an adequate trial at maximum dose.

 If there is >1 cause for nausea/vomiting you may need >1 drug.

Route of administration:
- For prophylaxis of nausea and vomiting—use po medication
- For established nausea or vomiting—consider a parenteral route e.g. syringe driver (p.185)—persistent nausea may ↓ gastric emptying and drug absorption. Once symptoms are controlled consider reverting to a po route.

Common side effects of anti-emetics:
- *Haloperidol and metoclopramide*—restlessness and/or urge to move (akathisia) or parkinsonian effects (e.g. stiffness, tremor)
- *Cyclizine*—anti-cholinergic effects e.g. dry mouth, blurred vision, urinary retention
- *Levomepromazine*—sedation at doses >6.25mg bd
- *Prokinetic drugs* (e.g. metoclopramide, domperidone)—use with care if bowel obstruction is suspected—may ↑ gut colic/worsen vomiting
- *Granisetron and ondansetron*—associated with constipation and headache.

Non-drug measures: Don't forget non-drug measures to ↓ nausea:
- Avoidance of food smells and unpleasant odours
- Relaxation/diversion/anxiety management
- Acupressure/acupuncture.

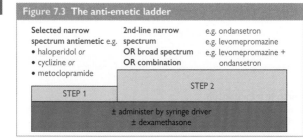

Figure 7.3 The anti-emetic ladder

Table 7.3 Causes of vomiting and choice of anti-emetic

Mechanism of vomiting	Anti-emetic
Drug/toxin-induced or metabolic e.g. hypercalcaemia	Haloperidol (1.5–5mg nocte). Levomepromazine 6.25mg nocte. If persistent nausea due to opioids, consider changing opioid.
Chemotherapy/ radiotherapy	Granisetron (1mg bd) or ondansetron (8mg bd po or 16mg od PR)—chemotherapy or radiotherapy-induced vomiting. Haloperidol 1.5–5mg nocte—radiotherapy-induced vomiting. Dexamethasone 4–8mg daily po/SC—often given as part of a chemotherapy regime. Metoclopramide 20mg qds.
Intra-cranial pressure	Dexamethasone 4–16mg/d. Cyclizine 50mg bd/tds (or 150mg/d. via syringe driver).
Anxiety, fear, or pain	Benzodiazepines e.g. diazepam 2–10mg/d. or midazolam sc. Cyclizine 50mg bd/tds. Levomepromazine 6–25mg/d.
Motion/position	Cyclizine 50mg tds po/SC/IM. Hyoscine po (300mcg tds) or transdermally (1mg/72h). Prochlorperazine po (5mg qds) or buccal (3–6mg bd).
Gastric stasis*	Domperidone 10mg tds or metoclopramide 10mg tds (particularly if multi-factorial with gastric stasis and a central component).
Gastric irritation	Stop the irritant if possible e.g. stop NSAIDs. Proton pump inhibitors e.g. lansoprazole 30mg od or omeprazole 20mg od. Antacids. Misoprostol 200mcg bd—if caused by NSAIDS.
Constipation	Laxatives/suppositories/enemas.
Intestinal obstruction	Refer for surgery if appropriate. Cyclizine, haloperidol, or levomepromazine. Dexamethasone 4–8mg/d—antiemetic and ↓ obstruction. If vomiting cannot be controlled consider referral for venting gastrostomy or antisecretory agents (e.g. octreotide).
Cough induced	📖 p.170
Unknown cause	Cyclizine 50mg tds or 150mg/d. via syringe driver. Levomepromazine 6–25mg/d. Dexamethasone 4–8mg daily po/SC. Metoclopramide 10–20 mg tds/qds po.

* vomits of undigested food without nausea soon after eating.

173

🅸 Drugs with anti-muscarinic effects (e.g. cyclizine) antagonize prokinetic drugs (e.g. metoclopramide)—if possible, don't use concurrently.

Other GI problems

Ascites: Free fluid in the peritoneal cavity. Common in ovarian cancer (50% patients) and GI cancer. Presents with abdominal distention. Examination reveals shifting dullness to percussion ± fluid thrill.

Management: Depending on clinical state consider referring for radio- or chemotherapy if appropriate *or* treat symptoms:

- Give analgesia for discomfort
- Refer for paracentesis and/or peritoneo-venous shunt
- Try diuretics—furosemide 20–40mg od and/or spironolactone 100–400mg od. May take a week to produce maximal effect.
  ⓘ monitor albumin level—if low, diuretics make ascites worse
- Dexamethasone 2–4mg daily may help—discontinue if not effective
- 'Squashed stomach syndrome'—try prokinetics e.g. domperidone or metoclopramide 10mg tds.

Constipation: Constipation is passage of hard stools less frequently than the patient's own normal pattern. It is a very common symptom. Causes—Table 7.4. Occult presentations are common in the very elderly and frail and include:

- Confusion
- Urinary retention
- Abdominal pain
- Overflow diarrhoea
- Loss of appetite
- Nausea and/or vomiting.

⚠ Constipation can herald spinal cord compression (📖 p.90). If suspected do a full neurological examination.

Table 7.4 Causes of constipation	
Malignancy	Colonic, ovarian, and uterine tumours.
Pain	Anal fissure, perianal abscess.
Benign colorectal disease	Diverticular disease, distal proctitis, anterior mucosal prolapse, benign stricture, intussusception, volvulus.
Endocrine/metabolic	Hypercalcaemia, hypothyroidism, DM with autonomic neuropathy.
Drugs	Opioids, antacids containing calcium or aluminium, antidepressants, iron, diuretics, antiparkinsonian medication, antimuscarinics e.g. phenothiazines, hyoscine, octreotide, anticonvulsants, antihistamines, calcium antagonists.
Other	Immobility, weakness (inability to ↑ intra-abdominal pressure), old age, poor diet, poor fluid intake, ↑ fluid loss (e.g. vomiting, diarrhoea, fever).

Management:

- Pre-empt constipation by putting everyone at risk (e.g. patients on opioids) on regular aperients
- Treat reversible causes e.g. give analgesia if pain on defecation, alter diet, ↑ fluid intake
- Treat with regular stool softener (e.g. lactulose) ± regular bowel stimulant (e.g. senna) or a combination drug (e.g. co-danthrusate). Titrate dose against response
- If that is ineffective consider adding rectal measures. If soft stools and lax rectum—try bisacodyl suppositories (🛈 must come into direct contact with rectum); if hard stools—try glycerol suppositories—insert into the faeces and allow to dissolve
- If still not cleared refer to the district nurse for lubricant ± high-phosphate (stimulant) enema (usually act in ~20min)
- Once cleared leave on a regular aperient with instructions to ↑ aperients if constipation recurs.

Diarrhoea: Clarify what the patient/carer means by diarrhoea. Less common than constipation but can be distressing for the patient and difficult for the carer—especially if incontinence results.

Management:

- ↑ fluid intake—small amounts of clear fluids frequently.
- Screen for infection (including pseudomembranous colitis if diarrhoea after a course of antibiotics) and treat if necessary.
- Ensure no overflow diarrhoea 2° to constipation
- Ensure no excessive/erratic laxative use
- Ensure no other medication is causing diarrhoea
- Consider giving aspirin (300–600mg tds)—↓ intestinal electrolyte and water secretion caused by prostaglandins. May particularly help with radiation-induced diarrhoea
- Consider ondansetron 4mg tds for radiotherapy-induced diarrhoea
- Consider giving pancreatic enzyme supplements e.g. Creon® 25,000 tds before meals if fat malabsorption (e.g. 2° to pancreatic carcinoma)
- Otherwise treat symptomatically with codeine phosphate 30–60mg qds or loperamide 2mg tds/qds
- Refer to palliative care if unable to control symptoms.

Further information:

European Journal of Palliative Care Campbell C Controlling malignant ascites (2001) **8** (5): 187–191.

Palliative Medicine Stephenson & Gilbert The development of clinical guidelines on paracentesis for ascites related to malignancy (2002) **16** (3): 213–218.

Doyle *et al. Oxford Textbook of Palliative Medicine* (2005) OUP ISBN: 0198566980

Skin care

Radiotherapy: All patients undergoing radiotherapy should be advised of the following. This advice applies to the area being treated including both the entry and the exit sites.

Washing:
- Use warm tepid water with unperfumed soap
- Do not use perfumed products
- Do not use a wash cloth
- Use a soft towel to pat the area dry
- Do not apply perfume, aftershave, or deodorant to treatment fields.

Hair removal:
- Use an electric shaver instead of a wet razor when shaving the face
- Do not shave other areas if they are in the treatment field.

Swimming: Chlorinated water can dry the skin and should usually be avoided.

Generally:
- Avoid direct application of heat or cold to the area
- Try to reduce all friction to the affected area
- Use of a mild detergent to wash clothes to be worn next to the skin to reduce irritation
- Avoid use of adhesive tape in irradiated field
- Avoid sun exposure
- Use sun screen of at least factor 15 for 1y after treatment
- Do not remove the skin markings which are applied by the radiotherapy department.

Management: See Table 7.5.

Bed sores:
- Owing to pressure necrosis of the skin
- Immobile patients are at high risk—especially if frail ± incontinent.
- Likely sites of pressure damage—shoulder blades, elbows, spine, buttocks, knees, ankles, and heels
- Bed sores heal slowly in terminally ill patients and are a source of discomfort and stress for both patients and carers (who often feel guilty that a pressure sore is a mark of poor care)
- If at risk refer to the district nurse or palliative care nursing team for advice on prevention of bed sores—protective mattresses and cushions, incontinence advice, advice on positioning and movement
- Warn carers to make contact with the district nurse or palliative care nursing team if a red patch does not improve 24h after relieving the pressure on the area
- Treat any sores that develop aggressively and admit if not resolving.

Table 7.5 Managing post-radiotherapy skin reactions

RTOG score*	Description	Appearance of skin	Treatment
0	Normal	Normal	Aqueous cream bd to delay onset of reaction. Normal washing as per guidelines.
1	Faint erythema	Skin slightly pink or red	Aqueous cream to soothe and moisturize tds or prn.
2A	Tender or bright erythema (dry desquamation)	Skin red, dry and scaly—some itch and tingling	Frequent aqueous cream (qds or prn). Diprobase cream or soft white paraffin (avoid excess build-up). Hydrocortisone cream may be used sparingly on itchy areas. Review use after 7d.—discontinue if the skin breaks.
2B	Patchy moist desquamation, oedema	Skin inflamed with patches of epidermis broken down and moist	Apply Hydrogel dressings to moist areas with appropriate secondary dressing e.g. surgipad or foam dressing. Apply aqueous cream to other parts of the field.
3	Confluent moist desquamation	Epidermis blisters and sloughs, underlying dermis is exposed and sore. Oozing of serous fluid	Apply Hydrogel or foam dressing suitable for the amount of exudate. Review frequently. Swab and treat with oral antibiotics (e.g. flucloxacillin 500mg qds) if any signs of infection.
After Radiotherapy	Reaction may continue for several weeks after treatment. Continue with use of aqueous creams until skin returns to normal. If RTOG* 2B/3 apply principles of moist wound healing as above or (if patient is not allergic to silicone) a silicone dressing. If infection is suspected apply silver impregnated dressings or silver sulfadiazine cream (Flamazine®).		

* RTOG stands for radiotherapy and oncology group.

Wound care:

- Large wounds can have major impact on quality of life
- Patients with advanced disease have major risk factors for development and poor healing of wounds—immobility, poor nutrition, skin infiltration ± breakdown due to malignancy
- Skin infiltration causing ulceration or fungating wounds can be particularly distressing.

Management: The primary aim is comfort. Healing is a secondary aim and may be impossible. Always involve the district nurse and/or specialist palliative care nursing team early. Many hospitals also have wound care specialist nurses who are invaluable sources of advice.

Specific management problems: See Table 7.6.

Body image: Odour, obvious dressings, facial disfigurement, and asymmetry can result in altered body image. As a result, patients may become socially isolated and experience difficulties in their relationships with their relatives/friends—including sexual problems.

Management:

- Talk to the patient and carers—give information and explanation
- Empathetic listening is often therapeutic in itself
- Ensure dressings are as leak proof and/or odour proof as possible
- Tailor dressings to the patient e.g. if going to a social event, avoid bulky, or unsightly dressings
- Consider counselling and/or management of depression or anxiety associated with altered body image where necessary.

Methicillin-resistant Staphylococcus aureus (MRSA): Difficult to eradicate. If causing the patient problems—discuss management with the local microbiology team. In all cases, warn health-care professionals in contact with the patient and any health or social-care establishment the patient will visit that the patient is MRSA +ve so that appropriate precautions can be taken to prevent spread to other patients.

Further information:

NICE Pressure ulcer management (2005) ▯ www.nice.org.uk

Table 7.6 Common wound management problems

Problem	Management
Pain	Exclude infection.
	Ensure the dressing is comfortable.
	Limit frequency of dressing changes.
	Ensure adequate background analgesia.
	Consider additional analgesia if needed for dressing changes and/or topical opioids on the dressing.
Excessive exudate	Use high-absorbency dressings with further packing on top ± plastic pads to protect clothing.
	Change the top layer of the dressing as often as needed but avoid frequent changes of the dressing placed directly on the wound.
	Protect the surrounding skin with a barrier cream/spray.
Necrotic tissue	Use desloughing agents.
	Referral for surgical debridement may be necessary.
Bleeding	Prevent bleeding during dressing changes by
	• avoiding frequent dressing changes
	• using non-adherent dressings or dressings which liquefy and can be washed off (e.g. Sorbsan®) *and*
	• irrigating the wound with saline to remove dressings.
	If there is surface bleeding—put pressure on the wound; if pressure is not working try
	• Kaltostat®
	• adrenaline—1mg/ml or 1:1000 on a gauze pad, *or*
	• sucralfate liquid—place on a non-adherent dressing and apply firmly to the bleeding area.
	Consider referral for radiotherapy or palliative surgery (e.g. cautery).
Odour	Treat with systemic and/or topical metronidazole.
	Charcoal dressings can be helpful.
	Seal the wound e.g. with additional layer of cling film dressing.
	Try disguising the smell with deodorisers (e.g. Nilodor®) used sparingly on top of the dressing—short-term measure. In the long term the deodorant smell often becomes associated with the smell of the wound for the patient.
Infection	Usually chronic and localized.
	Irrigate the wound with warm saline or under running water in the shower/bath.
	If the surrounding skin is inflamed—swab the wound and send for M, C, & S then start oral antibiotics e.g. flucloxacillin 250–500mg qds or erythromycin 250–500mg qds.
	Alter antibiotics depending on sensitivities of the organisms grown.

The last 48 hours

It is notoriously difficult to predict when death will occur. Avoid the trap of predicting or making a guess unless absolutely pushed to do so. Talk in terms of 'days' or 'weeks'. For example:

'When we see someone deteriorating from week to week we are often talking in terms of weeks; when that deterioration is from day to day then we are usually talking in terms of days, but everyone is different.'

Symptoms and signs of death approaching:
- Day by day deterioration
- Gaunt appearance
- Profound weakness—needs assistance with all care, may be bedbound
- Difficulty swallowing medicines
- ↓ intake of food and fluids
- Drowsy or ↓ cognition—often unable to co-operate with carers.

Goals of treatment in the last 48h:
- Ensure patients are comfortable—physically, emotionally, and spiritually
- Make the end of life peaceful and dignified—what is dignified for one patient may not be for another—ask
- Support patients and carers so that the experience of death for those left behind is as positive as it can be.

Patients' wishes: Dying is a unique and special event for each individual. Helping to explore a patient's wishes about death and dying should not be a discussion left to the last 24h.

Advance directives/living wills: 📖 p.209

Different cultures: Different religious and cultural groups have different approaches to the dying process. It is important to be sensitive to cultural and religious beliefs. If in doubt ask a family member. You are more likely to cause offence by not asking than by asking.

Assessment of a patient's needs: Try to discover which problems are causing the patient/carers most concern and address those concerns where possible. Patients often under-report their symptoms and families/carers may misinterpret symptoms.

Physical examination: Keep examination to a minimum to avoid unnecessary interference. Check:
- Sites of discomfort/pain suggested by history or non-verbal cues
- Mouth
- Bladder and bowel.

Psychological assessment: Find out what the patient wants to know. Gently assessing how the patient feels about their disease and situation can shed light on their needs and distress.

Investigations: Any investigation at the end of life should have a clear and justifiable purpose (e.g. excluding a reversible condition where treatment would make the patient more comfortable). The need for investigations in the terminal stage of illness is minimal.

Talking about death and dying: Death is a taboo subject and few people feel comfortable discussing it—even though it is natural, certain, and happening all around us all the time.

Opening up discussion can be very liberating to patients who then may feel they are being given permission to talk about dying. Families do not like discussions about dying for fear that patients will 'give up'.

Sometimes the direct question 'Are you worried about dying?' is the most appropriate. Often patients' biggest fears are groundless and reassurance can be given. Where reassurance cannot be given it is helpful to break the fear down into constituent parts and try to sort out those aspects you can deal with.

Common fears:

- *Fears associated with symptoms* e.g. pain will escalate to agony; breathing will stop if the patient falls asleep
- *Emotional fears* e.g. increasing dependence on family. 'It would be better if I was out of the way.'
- *Past experience* e.g. past contact with patients who died with unpleasant symptoms
- *Preferences about treatment or withholding treatment* e.g. 'What if nobody listens to me or takes my wishes seriously?'
- *Fears about morphine* e.g. 'Isn't that the stuff Dr. Shipman used?'
- *Death and dying*—fears of being dead and the process of dying need to be differentiated.

Review of medication:
- Comfort is the priority. Stop unnecessary medication
- Continue analgesia, antiemetics, anxiolytics/antipsychotics, and anticonvulsants
- Diabetes can be managed with short-acting insulin as needed
- Consider alternative routes of drug administration (e.g. syringe driver, patches)
- Explain changes to relatives/carers.

Symptom control: Dying patients tolerate symptoms very poorly because of their weakness. Nursing care is the mainstay of treatment. GPs do have a role though:
- Ensure new problems don't develop e.g. ensure use of appropriate mattresses and measures to prevent bed sores
- Treat specific symptoms e.g. dry mouth
- Think ahead—discuss treatment options which might be available later e.g. use of a syringe driver, buccal, PR, or transcutaneous preparations to deliver medication when/if the oral route is no longer possible, use of strong analgesia that may also have a sedative effect
- Ensure there is a clear management plan agreed between the medical and nursing team and the patient/family members. Anticipate probable needs of the patient so that immediate response can be made when the time comes—define clearly what should be done in the event of a symptom arising/worsening; ensure drugs or equipment that may be needed are in the home.

Referral to specialist palliative care services: Ideally involve specialist palliative care services before the terminal phase is reached. Referral in the terminal phase is appropriate when:
- One or more distressing symptoms prove difficult to control
- There is severe emotional distress
- There are dependent children and/or elderly vulnerable relatives involved.

Terminal anguish and spiritual distress:
- Characterized by overwhelming distress
- Often related to unresolved conflict, guilt, fears, or loss of control.

Anxiety can be increased if:
- Patients are unaware of the diagnosis, but feel people are lying to them
- They have certain symptoms such as breathlessness, haemorrhage, and constant nausea or diarrhoea
- Weak religious conviction—convinced believers and convinced non-believers have less anxiety
- There are young dependant children or other dependant relatives
- Patients have unfinished business to attend to, such as legal affairs.

Action: Empathic listening can itself be therapeutic. Talk to the patient, if possible, about dying and try to break down fears into component parts. Address those fears that can be dealt with. As a last resort, and after discussion with the patient (where possible) and/or relatives, consider sedation (see terminal restlessness/agitation).

Advice for patients: Patient experiences

Not wanting to be a burden:
'I don't want to be a burden to my family, that is something that's definitely out of order as far I'm concerned. I've seen other families that have endeavoured to cope with situations of that type when they couldn't and it practically destroyed the family.'

Choosing a place to die:
'I go back to my wife who died from cancer. One of the things she said to me was, 'I know I'm dying but I want to die in my own home.' And my response was, 'If we can manage to bring that wish to fulfilment we will do that.' And with the help of my 2 daughters and the local community nurses and the doctor, we managed to achieve that. It was hard work. It was very emotional but we managed to carry out her last wish.'

'I think if the cancer got bad I would like to go to a hospice. My husband is not terribly practical when it comes to looking after someone who is very ill and I think that I would like, if it came to it, I think I'd like to be in a hospice where they control the pain for you, look after you.'

Worries about death and dying:
'Again I don't know from the doctors what is likely to happen apart from they say I will just get weaker and weaker and as more pain occurs in the bones then I will be given more painkiller.'

'My biggest problem with thinking about death is not the actual dying because I can envisage that as going to sleep and not knowing anything about it like you go in for surgery. You have the anaesthetic and you're gone and you know nothing about it and you just don't wake up. I think of death like that.'

'What worries me is what's going to happen before [death], particularly with cancer because you hear so much about the pain. I've experienced pain, I've had the pain in this breast so I have experienced pain and that side of it does worry me in wondering how I would cope with it.'

Acceptance of dying:
'Everybody is so different. Some people can shout, some people can scream, some people are quiet, it's very different, difficult. But acceptance is a great thing. It heals the mind. You know, you didn't bring it on yourself. You didn't make yourself sick. It comes on. You don't know why. So, that's all I can say because that's all I can get from it. I accept it.'

'Life is a mixture of all sorts of things. There are sad moments and there are moments when things have gone wrong and there are things when you can be upset and angry about things, but find the positives. And rejoice in those positives and rejoice in the life that you've had. Celebrate the life that you've had and come to terms with the fact that it will ultimately end. The only difference is that you now know and some people . . . well it comes to an end and they don't know about it.'

Terminal restlessness: *Causes:*

- *Pain/discomfort*—urinary retention, constipation, pain which the patient cannot tell you about, excess secretions in throat
- *Opioid toxicity*—causes myoclonic jerking. The dose of morphine may need to be ↓ if a patient becomes uraemic
- *Biochemical causes*—↑ Ca^{2+}, uraemia—⚠ if it has been decided not to treat abnormalities DON'T check for them
- *Psychological/spiritual distress.*

Management:

- Treat reversible causes e.g. catheterization for retention, hyoscine to dry up secretions
- If still restless, treat with a sedative. This does NOT shorten life but makes the patient and any relatives in attendance more comfortable.

Suitable drugs: haloperidol 1–3mg tds po; chlorpromazine 25–50mg tds po; diazepam 2–10mg tds po, midazolam (10–100mg/24h via syringe driver or 5mg stat), or levomepromazine (50–150mg/24h via syringe driver or 6.25mg stat).

Excessive respiratory secretion (death rattle): Noisy, moist breathing. Rarely distresses patients but can be very distressing for relatives in attendance.

Management:

- Reassure relatives that the patient is not suffering or choking
- Try repositioning and/or tipping the bed head down (if possible) to reduce the noise
- Treat prophylactically—it is easier to prevent secretions forming than remove accumulated secretions.

Suitable drugs:

- Glycopyrronium—non-sedative—give 200 mcg SC stat and review after 1h If effective, give 200 mcg every 4h by SC injection or 0.6–1.2mg/24h via syringe driver
- Hyoscine hydrobromide—sedative in high doses—give 400 mcg SC stat and review response after 30min. If effective, give 400–600 mcg 4–8 hourly or 0.6–2.4mg/24h via syringe driver. If the patient is conscious and respiratory secretions are not too distressing, it may be more appropriate to use a transdermal patch (Scopaderm TTS® 1.5mg over 3d) or sublingual tablets (Kwells®). Dry mouth is a side effect.

Terminal breathlessness: Distressing symptom for patients/carers.

Management: Support carers in attendance and explain management

- Diamorphine or morphine: dose depends on whether the patient is being converted from oral morphine (or an alternative opioid), to diamorphine. If no previous opioid, start diamorphine 5mg/24h SC. If previously on oral morphine, divide the total 24h dose by three to obtain the 24h SC dose of diamorph. ↑ dose slowly as needed
- Midazolam 5–10mg/24h SC
- If sticky secretions—try nebulized saline ± physiotherapy.

Syringe drivers: Although drugs can usually be administered by mouth to control the symptoms of terminal illness, occasionally that is not possible. Portable syringe drivers give a continuous subcutaneous infusion and can provide good control of symptoms with little discomfort or inconvenience to the patient.

Indications:
- The patient is unable to take medicines by mouth owing to nausea and vomiting, dysphagia, severe weakness, or coma
- There is bowel obstruction and further surgery is inappropriate
- The patient does not want to take regular medication by mouth.

Drugs which can be used in syringe drivers:

Indication	Drugs
Nausea and vomiting	Haloperidol 2.5–10mg/24h
	Levomepromazine 5–200mg/24h (causes sedation in 50%)
	Cyclizine 150mg/24h (may precipitate if mixed with other drugs)
	Metoclopramide 30–100mg/24h
	Octreotide 300–600 mcg/24h (consultant supervision)
	Hyoscine hydrobromide 20–60mg/24h
Respiratory secretions	Hyoscine hydrobromide 0.6–2.4mg/24h
	Glycopyrronium 0.6–1.2mg/24h
Restlessness and confusion	Haloperidol 5–15mg/24h
	Levomepromazine 50–200mg/24h
	Midazolam 20–100mg/24h (and fitting)
Pain control	Diamorphine—a third to a half of the total daily morphine dose

Mixing drugs in syringe drivers: Provided there is evidence of compatibility, drugs can be mixed in syringe drivers. Diamorphine can be mixed with:

- Cyclizine
- Hyoscine hydrobromide
- Hyoscine butylbromide
- Midazolam
- Dexamethasone
- Levomepromazine
- Haloperidol
- Metoclopramide.

Common problems with syringe drivers:
- *If the syringe driver runs too slowly:* Check it is switched on; check the battery; check the cannula is not blocked
- *If the syringe driver runs too quickly:* Check the rate setting
- *Injection site reaction:* If there is pain or inflammation, change the injection site.

🔵 Subcutaneous infusion solution should be monitored regularly both to check for precipitation (and discoloration) and to ensure the infusion is running at the correct rate.

⚠ Incorrect use of syringe drivers is a common cause of drug errors.

Chapter 8

Benefits and legal aspects of care in the community

Pensions and benefits

Retirement pension: A state retirement pension is currently payable to women aged $\geq$ 60y and men aged $\geq$65y—even if still working. Entitlement age will rise to 65y for women between 2010 and 2020 (affects those born April 1950 to April 1955). Claim forms should be received automatically—if not request one through the local Jobseeker Plus office. Pensions are taxable.

Basic pension: Flat rate amount—different for single people and married couples. If not enough National Insurance (NI) contributions have been paid, amounts may $\downarrow$. >80y a higher rate is payable which is not dependant on NI contributions.

Increase for dependants: Paid if:
- The claimant's spouse is <60y. and earns under a set amount / does not receive certain other benefits
- The claimant has children (if claim made before April 2003).

 If hospitalized, retirement pension is payable for 1y at full rate. After 12 mo, basic pension is $\downarrow$.

Pension Credit: Apply on form PC1 ☎ 0800 991 234

Guarantee credit: $\geq$60y and income below the '*appropriate amount*'. Appropriate amount varies according to circumstances. Capital (excluding value of own home) >£6000 is deemed to count as income at the rate of £1/wk/£500 capital. Confers automatic eligibility for housing benefit, community tax benefit, and social fund payments.

Savings credit: $\geq$65y and income >savings credit starting point—currently >£167/wk for a single person or >£245 if one of a couple. Depends on level of income and circumstances.

Other benefits just for pensioners:
- *Free colour TV license:* All pensioners >75y
- *Winter fuel payment:* Annual payment to all pensioners >60y

Home Responsibilities Protection (HRP): Scheme which protects Basic State Pension for people who don't work or have low income and are caring for someone. www.thepensionservice.gov.uk

Christmas bonus: One-off payment made to people receiving a retirement pension or income support a few weeks before Christmas.

Cold Weather Payment: p. 182

Free prescriptions: All patients with cancer are dentitled to free prescriptions wherever they live in the UK. In England a MedEx form must be completed by the patient and GP/specialist and sent to the NHS Business Service Authority

Benefits for:

Bereavement benefits: Payable to men and women whose spouses have died—including civil partnership but co-habitation does not qualify except in Scotland. Claims can be made on forms available from Benefits offices or on-line via ⊞ www.jobcentreplus.gov.uk. *Benefits available:*

Bereavement payment: Lump sum payable if spouse has paid enough National Insurance contributions, or death was caused by employment, and the recipient is below state pension age at the time of the death. Claim <12mo. after death.

Widowed parent's allowance: Paid to widows/widowers with children or if pregnant.

Bereavement allowance: Paid for 52wk from the date of bereavement for spouses >45y old, not bringing up children and under retirement age.

Funeral payment: Table 8.1, 📖 p. 192

War pensions For people injured whilst serving in the armed forces and their dependants (if injury caused or hastened death). Administered by the Veterans Agency, Ministry of Defence. No time limit for claims.

War pensions scheme for ex-Service personnel whose injuries, wounds and illnesses arose prior to 6th April 2005. Includes War Disablement Pension and may meet the costs of some medical treatment.

War widows and widowers' pensions for spouses/civil partners of Service/ex-Service personnel if death occurred in service, or if the deceased was in receipt of a high rate War Disablement Pension with Unemployability Supplement or a War Pensions Constant Attendance Allowance.

Armed Forces Compensation Scheme (AFCS) provides benefits for illness, injury or death caused by service on or after 6th April 2005. Time limit is 5y from the event, from the time when medical advice was first sought or after retirement—whichever is soonest. There is an exceptions list for late onset conditions. Provides:
- Lump sum for significant illnesses/injuries—15 levels of award
- Tax-free Guaranteed Income Payment (GIP) for life for injuries at the higher tariff levels (1-11) to compensate for loss of earnings capacity
- Guaranteed Income Payment for Survivor's (SGIP) where an attributable death occurs

Further information
The Pension Service ⊞ www.thepensionservice.gov.uk
Pensions Advisory Service (TPA) ☎ 0845 601 2923
⊞ www.pensionsadvisoryservice.org.uk
Citizens Advice Bureau ⊞ www.adviceguide.org.uk
Veterans Agency ☎ 0800 169 22 77 ⊞ www.veterans-uk.info

Table 8.1 Benefits for people with low income

	Eligibility	How to apply	Benefits gained
Income Support (IS)	• ≥16y and <60y • Low income, <£8000 in savings (£16000 if in residential care) and not in receipt of JSA. • <16h paid work/wk (and partner <24h/wk)	Form A1 from local Job-centre plus office. Or online at 🖳 www.jobcentreplus.gov.uk	**Money**—depends on circumstances **Other benefits**—housing benefit, community tax benefit, health benefits and social fund payments. Children <5y. and pregnant women—free milk and vitamins. Children >5y.—free school meals and, in some areas, uniform grants. **Christmas bonus**— 📖 p.194
JobSeekers Allowance (JSA)	• ≥19y and <60y (women) or <65y (men). • Unemployed or working <16h / wk. • Capable of and available for work • Have a JobSeekers agreement that contracts the recipient to actively seek work.	Apply by visiting local Job-Centre plus office or online at 🖳 www.jobcentreplus.gov.uk	**Contributions-based JobSeekers allowance**—can claim for up to 26wk. Age-dependent fixed weekly pay-ment. **Income-based JobSeekers allowance**—allowance dependent on circumstances. Entitles claimants to same benefits as income support (see above). **Hardship payments**—available to people disallowed JSA.
Child Tax Credit (CTC)	• Age ≥16y and • Responsible for ≥1 child (<16y or 16-19y and in full time education). • Family income <£50,000 pa.	Apply to the Tax Office ☎ 0845 300 3900 🖳 www.hmrc.gov.uk	**Tax credits:** Family element—credit for any family eligible –i if there is a child <1y old in the family. Child element—credit for each individual child in the family— ↑ if the child is disabled / severely disabled.

	Eligibility	How to apply	Benefits gained
Working Tax Credit (WTC)	• Age ≥16y, working ≥16h/wk. and responsible for a child (<16y or 16–19y in full time education) • Age ≥16y, working ≥16h/wk and has a disability • Age ≥50y, working ≥16h/wk and has started work after ≥6mo of receiving 1 of certain benefits. • Age ≥25y and working ≥30h/wk..	Apply to the Tax Office ☎ 0845 300 3900 🖳 www.hmrc.gov.uk	**Tax credits**—depends on adding together elements: • Basic element—paid to everyone entitled to WTC • Second adult element • Lone parent element • Working >30h/wk. (can combine both parents if have children). • Disability (if working >16h/wk.) • Severe disability (if working >16h/wk.) • Aged ≥50y and in receipt of certain benefits before resuming work. • Childcare—up to 70% childcare costs
Health Benefits	**Automatic entitlement:** • >60 or <16y of age or 16–18y of age in full time education • Patient or family receiving: IS, income-based JSA or Pension Credit Guarantee Credit • Patients/families receiving Working Tax Credit or Child Tax Credit who have a valid NHS Tax Credit Exemption Certificate (should be supplied automatically) **By application:** • Low income *and* • Savings <£8000	If automatic exemption, no need to claim. If not, claim using form HC1 available from pharmacies, GP surgeries and local Jobcentre plus offices.	Free: • Prescriptions • NHS dentistry • NHS eye tests and glasses, • NHS wigs and fabric supports • Travel to hospital, • Milk and vitamins for pregnant and breast-feeding women, and children <5y

Table 8.1 Continued

Table 8.1 Continued

	Eligibility	How to apply	Benefits gained
Housing Benefit	Low income, living in rented housing. *Exclusions:* Full time students without dependants, people in residential care or with savings >£16,000.	Via local authority	Pays rent for up to 60wk. Then need to reapply.
Council Tax Benefit and Second Adult rebate	• **Council tax benefit:** Low income. Exclusions as for housing benefit. • **Second adult rebate:** Payable if someone who lives with you is aged >18y, does not pay rent or council tax and has low income. • **Council tax reduction:** If single occupier or disabled. • **Disregarded occupants:** Certain people including students, carers and children, are not counted in calculating the number of people living at a property.	Via local authority	**Council tax benefit :** pays council tax. **Council tax reductions:** • single occupier—25% discount • all disregarded occupants—50% • disabled—reduction to next lowest council tax band.
The 6 Social Fund payments	• **Crisis loan**—anyone except students and people in residential care can apply. • **Budgeting loan**—for large purchases. Must receive IS, pension credit or income-based JSA. • **Funeral Payments**—Must receive low income benefit and be responsible for the funeral. • **Cold weather payments**—average temperature <0°C for ≥7d. Must receive IS, pension credit or income-based JSA and live with a pensioner, child <5y or disabled person. • **Maternity grant** • **Community care grant**— p.195	Cold weather payments—should be automatic. All others claim via local Jobcentre plus offices or www.jobcentreplus.gov.uk	• **Crisis loan**—up to £1000—interest free loan repayable when crisis finished over 78wk. • **Budgeting loan**—as crisis loan • **Funeral expenses**—sum towards cost of funeral—usually does not cover full expenses. • **Cold weather payments**—£8.50/wk.

Table 8.2 **Benefits for disability and illness**

	Eligibility	How to apply	Amount
Statutory Sick Pay	• Employee age ≥16y and <65y • Incapable of work due to sickness or disability • Earning ≥ NI lower earnings limit • Unable to work ≥4d and <28wk (inc. days when would not normally work). • Those ineligible may be eligible for ESA or maternity allowance	Notify employer of ill-ness—self-certification (SC2) for first 7d; Med 3 after that time (📖 p.207)	£75.40 / wk. Some employers have more generous arrangements. Paid through normal pay mechanisms.
Employment and Support Allowance (ESA)	• Age ≥16y and <60y (woman) or <65y (man) • Not entitled to statutory sick pay • Unable to work due to sickness or disability—SC1 certifica-tion for first 7d then Med3 certifica-tion until work capability assessment (done <13wk into period of sickness/disability)—📖 p.207 • Not receiving income support, income based Job Seeker's Allowance or Pension Credit **2 types of ESA** • *Contributory ESA*—paid if sufficient NI contributions (unless unfit for work under the age of 20 (25 if in full time education) • *Income related ESA*—full rate is paid if savings ≤£16,000 and income is less than a minimum income; reduced rates may be payable if income is greater than this minimum amount	Claim from 🖥 www.jobcentreplus.gov.uk or ☎0800 055 6688 (text-phone: 0800 023 4888)	*First 3d*—no payment *Assessment phase* (>3d but <14wk). • <25y—up to £51.85 • ≥25y—up to £66.45 *Main phase* (≥14wk) • Work related activity group—up to £91.40 • Support group—up to £96.85 ❶ Figures are for a single person. Addi-tional payments may be available for dependants if receiving income-related ESA

❶ Incapacity Benefit—Since 27.10.2008, ESA has replaced Incapacity Benefit for new claims. Those people already receiving Incapacity Benefit will continue to do so at present.

Table 8.2 Continued

	Eligibility	How to apply	Amount
Disability Living Allowance (DLA)[v]	• Disability >3mo and expected to last >6 mo. more*. • <65y at time of application **Mobility Component** Help needed to get about outdoors • *Higher rate*—unable/virtually unable to walk (age >3y) • *Lower rate*—help to find way in unfamiliar places (age >5y) **Care Component** Help needed with personal care • *Lower rate*—attention/supervision needed for a significant proportion of the day or unable to prepare a cooked meal. • *Middle rate*—attention/ supervision throughout the day or repeated prolonged attention or watching over at night. *Higher rate*—24 hour attention / supervision day or terminal illness*	☎0800 882200 (0800 220674 in Northern Ireland) or Leaflet DLA A5DCS available from Post Offices or Using claim packs available at Citizen's Advice Bureau and social security offices or 🖥 www.direct. gov.uk	**Mobility Component** *Higher rate*—£49.85/wk *Lower rate*—£18.95/ wk **Care Component** *Higher rate*—£71.40/wk *Middle rate*—£47.80/wk *Lower rate*—£18.95/wk
Attendance Allowance (AA) [v]	• Disability >3mo and expected to last >6mo more*. • Aged ≥65y • Not permanently in hospital or accommodation funded by the local authority • Needs attention / supervision—higher rate if 24 hour care required/terminal illness*	☎0800 882200 (0800 220674 in Northern Ireland) or Leaflet AA A5DCS available from Post Offices or 🖥 www.direct.gov.uk	*Lower rate £47.80* *Higher rate £71.40 (for people who need day and night care or are terminally ill)*

[v] No need to receive help to apply. Not means tested.

*Terminal illness (not expected to live >6mo)—claim under Special Rules. Claims are processed much faster and the highest care rate is automatically awarded. GP or hospital specialist fills in form DS1500 to provide clinical information to support application (fee can be claimed).

Table 8.2 Continued

	Eligibility	How to apply	Amount
Community Care Grant	Receiving Income Support or income-based Jobseeker's allowance and: • want to re-establish or help the applicant or a family member stay in the community • ease exceptional pressure on the applicant or a family member. • to help with certain travel costs	Form SF300 from local social security offices or 🖥 www.dwp.gov.uk	Minimum payment £30. No maximum amount.
Disabled facilities grant	For work essential to help a disabled person live an independent life. Means tested.	Apply via local housing department.	Any reasonable application for funds is considered.
Carer's allowance	• Aged ≥16y; and • Spends ≥35h/wk caring for a person with a disability who is getting AA or constant attendance allowance or middle or higher rate care component of DLA; and • Earning ≤£95.00/wk After allowable expenses • Not in full time education	Ccmplete form in leaflet CAASDCS available from local social security offices or 🖥 www.direct.gov.uk	£53.90/wk *Plus* additions for dependants. 🔵 no new claims for dependent children have been accepted since April 2003)

🔵 *Severe disablement allowance is still paid to those who applied prior to April 2001*

Table 8.3 Mobility for elderly and disabled people		Local public transport schemes also exist	
	Eligibility	How to apply	Benefits gained
Blue Badge Scheme	Age >2y and ≥1 of the following: • War Pensioner's mobility supplement • Higher rate of the mobility component of DLA • Motor vehicle supplied by a Government Health department • Registered blind • Severe disability in both upper limbs preventing turning of a steering wheel • Permanent and substantial difficulty walking	Apply through local social services department. ℹ In most circumstances the disabled person does not have to be the driver. The badge should not be used if the disabled person is not in the car. 🖥 www.dft.gov.uk	Entitles holder to park: • in specified disabled spaces; • free of charge or time limit at parking meters or other places where waiting is limited • on single yellow lines for up to 3h (no time limit in Scotland)
Motability Scheme	• Higher rate mobility component of DLA or • War Pension Mobility Supplement ℹ Driver may be someone else.	Contact motability. Application guide available at 🖥 www.motability.co.uk	Registered Charity. Mobility payments can be used to lease or hire-purchase a car, powered scooter or wheelchair. Grants may also be available for advance payments, adaptations or driving lessons.
Road Tax Exemption	• Higher rate mobility component of DLA or • War Pension Mobility Supplement or • Person nominated as someone who regularly drives for a disabled person or • Certain types of powered invalid carriages	Usually received automatically. If not and claiming DLA ☎ 0845 7123456. If claiming War Pension ☎ 0800 1692277	Exemption from Road Tax.
Seatbelt exemption	Certain medical conditions e.g. colostomy	Medical practitioner must complete exemption certificate	Exemption from wearing seatbelt

Table 8.4 Adaptations and equipment for elderly and disabled people ● All purchases related to disability are VAT exempt.

	Eligibility	Applying	Benefits received
Wheelchairs	Anyone requiring a wheelchair(s) for >3mo. Short term loan of equipment is often available via the Red Cross.	Referral by GP or specialist to the wheelchair service centre. Directory of service centres is available at: 🖳 www.wheelchairmanagers.nhs.uk	Provision of suitable wheelchair. Vouchers enable disabled patients to purchase their chairs privately.
Occupational Therapy (OT) Assessment	All elderly or disabled people	Request a needs assessment by an occupational therapist via local social services department.	Enables provision of equipment and adaptations necessary to maintain an independent lifestyle
Disabled Living Centres / Disability Living Foundation	All elderly or disabled people	49 *Disabled Living Centres* in the UK—list available from 🖳 www.assist-uk.org *Disabled Living Foundation* 🖳 www.dlf.org.uk.	*Disabled Living Centres:* Look at and try out equipment with OTs on hand to advise. *Disabled Living Foundation:* Information on aids and adaptations
Telephone	People who have physical difficulty using the telephone or communication problems.	British Telecom produce a booklet "Communication solutions" obtainable from ☎0800 800150 or 🖳 www.bt.com If difficulty using a telephone directory register to use directory enquiries free ☎0800 5870195	Gadgets and services that make it easier for disabled or elderly people to use the telephone.
Alarm Systems	Any disabled or elderly person who is alone at times, at risk, and mentally capable of using an alarm system.	Arrange via local Social Services or Housing Department. Alternatively charities have schemes (Help the Aged -seniorlink ☎0808 800 6565; Age Concern—Aid-Call ☎0800 772266).	Enables a call for help when the 'phone cannot be reached.

Occupational illness

If a patient develops an occupational disease, a doctor is obliged to notify the employer in writing with the patient's consent. The doctor does not need to make a judgment about whether the disease is, in that particular case, caused by the occupation. Employers must then inform the Reporting of Injuries, Diseases and Dangerous Occurrences Regulations (RIDDOR) incident contact center (☎ 0845 300 99 23 ⌨ www.riddor.gov.uk). Self-employed patients must contact RIDDOR themselves.

Patients who do not give consent for the doctor to notify their employer may allow the doctor to inform the employer's occupational health department or RIDDOR directly instead.

Notifiable industrial cancers:
- Cancer of bronchus or lung caused by industrial exposure to carcinogens
- Primary carcinoma of the lung where there is accompanying evidence of silicosis
- Nasal or sinus cancer caused by occupational exposure to carcinogens (wood, fibreboard, nickel, and leather workers)
- Mesothelioma due to asbestos exposure
- Bladder cancer in plastic workers
- Cancers as a result of ionizing radiation.

ⓘ This is not a complete list—for a complete list see *RIDDOR: Information for doctors* available from ⌨ www.hse.gov.uk

---

Prescribed industrial disease: Disease for which benefit is paid if the applicant worked in a job for which that disease is 'prescribed' and it is likely that the employment caused the disease. Claims may be made at any time for occupational cancers. The list of prescribed diseases is similar to but *not* the same as the list of notifiable diseases.

Benefits that may be payable:

Industrial injuries disablement benefit: Available to employed earners for certain (prescribed) illnesses arising as a result of employment, even if the employee was either part or wholly to blame. This scheme covers virtually all forms of work.

Constant attendance allowance: Available for people so disabled they need constant care and attention and who are getting disablement benefit for disability assessed at 100%. His has four rates of benefit.

Exceptionally severe disablement allowance: Available for people who get constant attendance allowance at high rate and where need for attendance is likely to be permanent.

Making claims: Claiming through local Jobcentre plus or social security office. A full list of prescribed industrial diseases is also available from these places. Some claims can be made online ⌨ www.jobcentreplus.gov.uk

Further information:

RIDDOR Incident contact center ☎ 0845 300 99 23 ⌨ www.riddor.gov.uk

Compensation for workers disabled by lung disease:

Pneumoconiosis etc. (Workers' Compensation) Act 1979: This is for sufferers of certain industrial diseases caused by dust, irrespective of industry. If the patient has died, a dependant may claim. Sufferers must be unable to claim damages from the employers who caused the disease because they have ceased trading. The sufferer or dependants must not have brought a court action or received compensation from an employer in respect of the disease.

Diseases covered:
- Diffuse mesothelioma
- Pneumoconiosis (including silicosis, asbestosis, and kaolinosis)—except former coal industry workers who are covered by a separate scheme (below)
- Diffuse pleural thickening
- Primary lung cancer if accompanied by asbestosis or diffuse pleural thickening
- Byssinosis.

⚠ Sufferers should normally be in receipt of disablement benefit for the disease. Dependants can claim disablement benefit posthumously but there are time limits for the claim—if time barred, dependants can still make a claim.

Further information: ☎ 0800 279 23 22 🖳 www.jobcentreplus.gov.uk

Coal miners: Former coal industry workers suffering from pneumoconiosis, chronic bronchitis, and/or COPD are covered by a separate scheme administered on behalf of the Department of Trade and Industry (☎ 0114 203 4359).

Asbestos-related disease: Governmental compensation is changing and this may be available for people with pleural, pericardial, and peritoneal mesothelioma without definite occupational exposure.

Government: May NOT apply to non-employees
- Industrial injuries disablement benefit—next of kin can claim up to 6mo. posthumously
- War Disablement Pensions scheme—if exposure with as a result of work in the armed forces
- Pneumoconiosis etc. (Worker's Compensation) Act—above—if no claim can be made against the employer.

Courts:
- Claims are fought with difficulty. Expert legal advice from a lawyer specializing in asbestos compensation claims is essential
- Victims must establish their condition was caused by work and due to negligence on the part of their employers or someone else
- Sufferers or their dependants can make claims against a previous employer, the company responsible for their exposure (e.g. exposure due to living near an asbestos factory or exposure of a spouse due to washing clothes etc.) or the company's insurer
- Usually claims must be initiated <3y. after diagnosis of an asbestos-related disease.

Support of informal carers

In the UK there are 6 million informal carers. Most are relatives or friends of the person being cared for. Many are elderly with health problems themselves. There is good evidence their health suffers as a result of caring—52% report treatment for a stress-related illness since becoming a carer and 51% report being physically injured as a result of caring.

GPs and their primary care teams are often the first point of access for any help needed and 88% of carers have seen their GP in the past 12 mo. Carers see the GP as the professional most able to improve their lives but few GPs have had any training about their problems and 71% carers believe their GPs are unaware of their needs.

Physical help: Record whether a patient is a carer in their notes.
- *Practical advice on nursing skills*—ask distrct nurses to review
- *Advice on management*—specialist nurses (e.g. Macmillan nurses etc.) provide special expertise.
- *Additional help*—social services can provide home care. Voluntary organisations provide sitting services e.g. Crossroads schemes.
- *Home modification*—local authorities can arrange modifications. District nurses have access to equipment needed for nursing. The Red Cross loans commodes, wheelchairs etc.
- *Respite*—hospices, charity organisations and local authorities may provide day care (to give regular breaks each week) and respite care (for a week or more at a time).

Emotional support:
- *Self-help carers groups*—opportunity to share experiences with people in similar situations.
- *Always ask the carer how they are when visiting*—even if not your patient.
- *If the patient and / or carer have a religion, the clergy will often provide ongoing support.*
- *Maintain good lines of communication.* Treat the carer as a team member. Make sure you inform both carer and patient fully. Don't be short with a carer, patronising or impossible to contact.

Financial support: Many patients who have carers are entitled to Attendance Allowance or Disability Living Allowance (📖 p.194). If the patient is not expected to live >6mo. they are entitled to claim under Special Rules. This benefit is not means tested. Other benefits:
- *Low income*—Table 8.1, 📖 p.190
- *Given up work to look after the patient*—may be eligible for carers allowance—📖 p.195.
- *Substantial modification to home*—Council Tax may be payable at lower rate (consult local council).

GP services
- Try to identify carers e.g. scanning discharge summaries for patients with cancer, opportunistically
- Consider asking for written consent from the people cared for to share medical information about them with their carers

- Provide appointments for carers at times when they can attend. Consider offering home visits for the carer if unable to get to the sugery as a result of caring duties
- Offer carers an annual influenza vaccination
- Include carers as partners in care

The RCGP and Princess Royal Trust for carers have developed a self-assessment checklist and action guide for GP practices to help them to support carers. *Supporting carers: an action guide for general practitioners and their teams* is available from 🖳 www.carers.org

Social services assessment Every carer has a right to ask for a full assessment of their needs by the social services. Emergency planning is part of the carer's assessment.

Emergency planning Advise carers to make an emergency plan. Emergency plans are lodged on a database and the carer is provided with a card to carry with the emergency contact number printed on it.
- If carers have an unexpected crisis and cannot provide care, they can ring the emergency line with the knowledge that short-term replacement care will be available.
- Carers are advised to carry the cards with them in an obvious place (e.g. wallet or purse). In the event of mishap, this will alert that the person is a carer and allow the emergency plan to be activated.

Support organizations for carers
NHS Carers Direct ☎ 0808 802 0202 🖳 www.nhs.uk/carersdirect
Disability and carers service 🖳 www.direct.gov.uk/carers or www.direct.gov.uk/disability
Carers UK ☎ 0808 808 7777 🖳 www.carersuk.org
Princess Royal Trust for Carers ☎ 0844 800 4361
🖳 www.carers.org
Benefits Enquiry Line ☎ 0800 882200; 0800 243355 (minicom facility); 0800 441144 (for help with form completion)
Citizens Advice Bureau 🖳 www.adviceguide.org.uk
Age UK ☎ 0800 169 65 65 🖳 www.ageuk.org.uk
Counsel and Care ☎ 0845 300 7585 🖳 www.counselandcare.org.uk
Support organisations for the patient's condition

GP notes

Carer skills: A carer skills course has been developed by Caring with Confidence. Further information is available at 🖳 www.caringwithconfidence.net

---

GMS contract

Management 9	The practice has a protocol for the identification of carers and a mechanism for the referral of carers for social services assessment	3 points

Controlled drugs

Misuse of Drugs Act (1971) Controls manufacture, supply and possession of controlled drugs. Penalties for offences are graded according to perceived harmfulness of the drug into 3 classes:

- Class A: e.g. cocaine, diamorphine (heroin), methadone, LSD, D-lysergic acid diethylamide ecstasy.
- Class B: e.g. oral amphetamines, barbiturates, cannabis
- Class C: e.g. most benzodiazepines, androgenic and anabolic steroids

Misuse of Drugs Regulations (2001) Defines persons authorised to supply and possess CDs while carrying out their professions and describes the way in which this is to be done. 5 schedules of drug:

- Schedule 1: Drugs not used for medicinal purposes e.g. LSD. Possession and supply are prohibited except with special licence.
- Schedule 2: Drugs subject to full CD controls (written dispensing record, kept in locked container, CD prescription regulations) e.g. diamorphine, cocaine, pethidine.
- Schedule 3: Partial CD controls (as schedule 2 but no need to keep a register—some drugs subject to safe custody regulations) e.g. barbiturates, temazepam, meprobamate, buprenorphine.
- Schedules 4 and 5: Most benzodiazepines, anabolic and androgenic steroids, HCG, growth hormone, codeine. Controlled drug prescription requirements do not apply nor do safe custody requirements.

❶ Preparations in Schedules 2 and 3 are identified throughout the British National Formulary (BNF) by the symbol ▣ (controlled drug).

Controlled drugs register All health care professionals who hold personal stock of any Schedule 2 drugs must keep their own controlled drugs register, and they are personally responsible for keeping this accurate and up-to-date. Out-of-date drugs should be recorded and destroyed in the presence of an authorized witness (police, PCO official).

Writing prescriptions for controlled drugs: Any prescription for Schedule 2 and 3 controlled drugs (with the exception of temazepam) must contain the following details, written so as to be indelible:

- The patient's full name, address and age—if the patient is homeless, 'no fixed abode' is an acceptable address
- The patient's NHS (in Scotland, Community Health Index) number
- Name and form of the drug, even if only one form exists
- Strength of the preparation and dose to be taken
- The total quantity of the preparation, or the number of dose units, to be supplied in both words and figures e.g. 'Morphine sulphate 10 mg (ten milligram) tablets, one to be taken twice daily. Supply 60 (sixty) tablets, total 600 (six hundred) milligrams'
- Signature of the prescriber (must be handwritten) and date. It is good practice to include the GMC number of the prescriber as well.
- The address of the prescriber

❶ Apart from in exceptional circumstances, prescriptions for CDs in Schedules 2,3 & 4 should be limited to a supply of ≤30d treatment. The validity period of NHS and private prescriptions for Schedule 1, 2, 3 and 4 controlled drugs is restricted to 28 d. Schedule 2 and 3 drugs cannot be prescribed on repeat prescriptions or under repeat dispensing schemes.

Prescriber's responsibilities:
- To avoid creating dependence by unnecessarily introducing controlled drugs to patients.
- Careful monitoring to ensure the patient does not gradually ↑ the dose of drug to a point where dependence becomes more likely.
- To avoid being an unwitting source of supply for addicts. If you suspect an addict is going round surgeries with intent to obtain supplies, contact your PCO so that they can issue a warning to other practices.

Further information:

National Prescribing Centre (NPC) A guide to good practice in the management of controlled drugs in primary care (England) (2007) 🖳 www.npc.co.uk
Department of Health 🖳 www.dh.gov.uk/controlleddrugs
British National Formulary 🖳 www.bnf.org
Home Office Tackling Drugs: Changing lives 🖳 www.drugs.gov.uk

---

GP notes

Travelling with controlled drugs: For patients or doctors travelling abroad with schedule 2 or 3 drugs, an export license may be required. Further details are available from ☎ 020 7035 4848 or 🖳 www.drugs.gov.uk/drugs-laws/licensing/personal. Patient applications to the Home Office for an import/export licence for a controlled drug must be accompanied by a supporting letter from the prescribing doctor stating:
- the patient's name and address
- the quantities of drugs to be carried
- the strength and form in which the drugs will be dispensed
- the country of destination
- the dates of travel to and from the UK

⚠ For clearance to import the drug into the country of destination, it is advisable to contact the Embassy or High Commission of that country prior to departure.

Licensing of drugs

In the UK, the Medicines Act (1968) makes it essential for anyone who manufactures or markets a drug for which therapeutic claims are made, to hold a licence. The Licensing Authority, working through the Medicines and Healthcare Products Regulatory Agency (MHRA), can grant both Manufacturer's Licence and Marketing Authorisation (which allows a company to market and supply a product for specified indications). Although doctors usually prescribe according to the licensed indications, they are not obliged to.

Prescribing outside licence: There may be occasions when a doctor feels it is necessary to prescribe outside a drug's licence:

- *Generic formulations* for which indications are not described. The prescriber has to assume the indications are the same as for branded formulations
- *Use of well-established drugs for proven but not licensed indications,* e.g. amitriptyline for neuropathic pain. Commonly occurs in palliative care (25% of prescriptions affecting 66% of patients) and chronic pain management. Most cases applies to 'new' uses for 'old' drugs where it is uneconomic for the manufacturer to obtain a license
- *Use of drugs for conditions where there are no other treatments* (even if the evidence of their effectiveness is not well proven). This often occurs in secondary care when new treatments become accepted. GPs may become involved if a patient is discharged to the community and the GP asked to continue prescribing
- *Use of drugs for individuals not covered by their licensed indications.* Frequently occurs in paediatrics.

⚠ Before prescribing any medication (whether within or outside the licence) weigh risks against benefits. The more dangerous the medicine, and the flimsier the evidence-base for treatment, the more difficult it is to justify the decision to prescribe.

When prescribing licensed drugs for unlicensed indications:

- Inform patients and carers of what you are doing and why and obtain consent for the drug's use in that way
- Explain that the patient information leaflet (PiL) will not have information about the use of the drug in these circumstances
- Record in the patients notes your reasons for prescribing outside the licensed indications for the drug.

🚫 The person signing the prescription is legally responsible.

Use of established bodies of evidence: If prescribing off license, be able to justify your decision to use the drug in question. Established bodies of evidence can provide justification. Suitable sources include the following:

- Cochrane database
- Drugs and Therapeutics Bulletin
- British National Formulary
- Palliative Care Formulary
- Textbooks of palliative care and local palliative care guidelines.

Further information:

Drugs and Therapeutics Bulletin Prescribing unlicensed drugs or using drugs for unlicensed applications (1992) **30:** 97–9

European Journal of Anaesthesiology Cohen P Off-label use of prescription drugs: legal, clinical and policy considerations (1997) **14:** 231–50

Association of Palliative Medicine and Pain Society The use of drugs beyond licence in palliative care and pain management (2002)

Twycross et al. *Palliative Care Formulary 2* (2002—2nd edition) Radcliffe Medical Press ISBN:

Certifying fitness to work

Own occupation test: Applies to those claiming statutory sick pay for the first 28wk. of their illness. The doctor assesses whether the patient is fit to do their *own* job.

Work capability assessment: Assesses a patient on a variety of different mental and physical health dimensions for ability to work. Not diagnosis dependant. Applies to:
- everyone after 28wk incapacity
- those who do not qualify for the own occupation test from the start of their incapacity.

The following tests are performed in the first 13 wk of any claim for Employment and Support Allowance (ESA; 📖 p. 193):

Limited capability for work assessment: In most cases this takes the form of a medical examination assessing mental and physical ability to work. Groups who will not be considered unfit to work without medical examination include pregnant women, people with severe physical or learning disability, and those who are terminally ill.

Limited capability for work-related activity assessment: This is usually carried out at the same time as the medical examination and is used to place individuals into one of two groups on the basis of their ability to perform any work:
- *Work related activity group*—individuals are expected to take part in work-focused interviews with their personal advisers, and are provided with a range of support to help them to prepare for a return to work. Those refusing to participate will have their benefit reduced.
- *Support group*—for those who have an illness/disability that has a severe effect of their ability to work. These individuals are not expected to take part in any work related activity, but can choose to do so on a voluntary basis.

Work-focused health-related assessment: Only for those placed in the work-related activities group. It collects additional information about activities that individuals can do. It explores the individual's wishes and aspirations regarding work, and problems that the individual may face getting into work and/or staying in work. It also looks at ways to manage these difficulties and/or minimize them.

Private certificates: Some employers request private certificates in the first week of sickness absence. They should request this in writing. If the GP chooses to provide the service, s/he may charge, both for a private consultation and the provision of a private certificate. The company should accept full responsibility for all fees incurred by the patient.

Disability Discrimination Act 1995: Requires employers to make reasonable adjustments for an employee with a long term disability. In 2005 the scope of the Act was amended and expanded. It now covers individuals suffering from cancer from the point of diagnosis rather than from when their condition impinges on their ability to perform their activities of daily living. Advise patients to seek specialist advice.

Forms for certifying incapacity to work:

SC1—self-certification form for people not eligible to claim statutory sick pay who wish to claim ESA. Certify first 7d of illness. Available from local Jobcentre Plus offices and GP surgery.

SC2—as SC1 but for people who can claim statutory sick pay. Available from employer, local Jobcentre Plus offices and GP surgery.

Med 3—*Statement of Fitness for Work*—filled in by a GP or hospital doctor who knows the patient for periods of incapacity likely to be >7d. During the first 6mo of incapacity, Statements of Fitness for Work can only be issued for a maximum period of 3 mo. The doctor has two options:
* To indicate that the patient is unfit for work
* To indicate that the patient may be fit for work but only under certain circumstances —the GP may stipulate conditions which might allow return to work (e.g. allowing time off for ongoing treatment, adjusting work hours, or restricting work duties). The form gives space for the GP to record the patient's functional limitations and is designed to allow the employer to make adjustments to facilitate the employee's return to work.

ⓘ A Statement is not required to certify that a patient is fully fit to return to work without adjustments. If an employer requires such a statement, it should be requested as a private service.

The Statement of Fitness for work may be issued:
* on the day of your assessment of the patient (telephone consultations are acceptable)
* on a date after your assessment of the patient if you think that it would have been reasonable to issue a Statement on the day of your assessment of the patient
* after consideration of a report about the patient from another doctor or registered health care professional
* Only one Statement of Fitness for Work can be issued per patient per period of sickness. If mislaid reissue and mark 'duplicate'.

Further information:

Department of Work and Pensions. Statement of Fitness for Work: A guide for general Practitioners and other doctors
🖥 www.dwp.gov.uk/docs/fitnote-gp-guide.pdf
Disability Discrimination Act 🖥 www.direct.gov.uk/disability

Confirmation and certification of death

⚠ The death certification process in England and Wales is currently under review and is likely to change in the near future.

English law *does not* require a doctor
- To confirm death has occurred or that 'life is extinct'. A doctor is only required to certify what, in their opinion, was the cause
- To view the body of a deceased person. There is no obligation to see/examine a body before issuing a death certificate
- To report the fact that death has occurred.

English law *does* require the doctor who attended the deceased during the last illness to issue a certificate detailing the cause of death. Certificates are provided by the local Registrar of births, marriages and deaths.

Death in the community: A quarter of deaths occur at home.

Expected deaths: In all cases, advise to contact the undertakers and ensure the patient's own GP is notified.
- *Patient's home:* visit as soon as practicable
- *Residential/nursing home:* if possible the GP who attended during the patient's last illness should visit and issue a death certificate. The 'on-call' GP is often requested to visit. There is no statutory duty to do this but it is reassuring for the staff at the home and often necessary before staff are allowed to ask for the body to be removed.

Unexpected and/or 'sudden' death: If called, advise the attendant to call the emergency services. Visit and take a rapid history from any attendants. Then:
- Resuscitate if appropriate
- Report the death to the coroner—If any suspicious circumstances or circumstances of death are unknown/unclear—call the police.

Alternatively, if police or ambulance service is already in attendance and death has been confirmed, suggest the police surgeon is contacted.

Cremation: The Cremation Regulations (2008) require two doctors to complete a certificate to establish identity and that the cause of death is not suspicious before a person can be cremated. The person arranging the funeral may see the forms and pays a fee to each doctor. There are two parts:
- *Cremation 4:* Completed by the patient's usual medical attendant—usually his/her GP
- *Cremation 5:* Completed by another doctor who must have held full GMC registration (or equivalent) for ≥5y. and is not connected with the patient in any way nor directly connected with the doctor who issued *Cremation 4*—usually a GP from another practice.

⚠ Pacemakers, radioactive implants and certain internal fixator devices must be removed from the deceased before cremation can take place.

- Sudden or unexpected deaths
- Accidents and injuries
- Industrial diseases e.g. mesothelioma
- Service disability pensioners
- Deaths where the doctor has not attended within the past 14d.
- Deaths arising from ill treatment e.g. abuse, neglect, starvation, hypothermia.
- Cause of death unknown
- Deaths <24h after hospital admission
- Poisoning (chronic alcoholism and its sequelae are no longer notifiable)
- Medical mishaps (including anaesthetic complications, short- or long-term complications of operations, drugs—whether therapeutic or addictive)
- Abortions
- Prisoners
- Stillbirths (if there is doubt about whether the baby was born alive).

Notification of death to the coroner: The coroner can be contacted via the local police. Reporting to the coroner does not automatically entail a post-mortem. The coroner, once circumstances of death are clear, may advise the GP to tick and initial box A on the back of the certificate which advises the Registrar that no inquest is necessary. Deaths which *MUST* be reported to the coroner are listed in Box 8.1.

 In Scotland deaths are reported to a procurator fiscal. The list of reportable deaths is the same with the addition of deaths of foster children and the newborn.

Recording deaths at the practice: Death registers are useful. Routine communication of deaths to all members of the primary health-care team and other agencies involved with the care of that patient (e.g. hospital consultants, social services) avoids the embarrassing and distressing situation of ongoing appointments and contacts being made for that patient. Record the death in the notes of any relatives/partner registered with the practice.

Benefits available after a death:

- For widows/widowers: p.189
- Funeral payment: Table 8.1, p.192.

Advice for patients: Advice and support

Department of work and pensions (DWP)
- Leaflet D49: What to do after a death in England and Wales. Available from www.dwp.gov.uk/publications/dwp/2006/d49_april06.pdf
- Funeral payment: Information and online application form www.jobcentreplus.gov.uk

Scottish Executive What to do after a death in Scotland. Available from www.scotland.gov.uk/publications/2006/04/1209444010

Mental Capacity, consent and decisions

Mental capacity is the ability to take actions affecting daily life (e.g. when to get up, what to wear, what to eat) and/or make more major decisions (e.g. where to live, how to manage money).

Mental Capacity Act (2005): came into force in 2007 in England and Wales. Similar legislation applies elsewhere in the UK. It specifies who can take decisions on behalf of other people and allows people to plan ahead for a time when they may lack capacity. Five key principles:

- Every adult has the right to make decisions and must be assumed to have capacity to make them unless proved otherwise.
- Every adult must be given all possible help and support to make decisions, and to communicate those decisions where necessary, before s/he can be assumed to have lost capacity.
- Making an unwise decision does not mean that a person lacks capacity to make that decision.
- Anything done or any decision made on behalf of someone who lacks capacity must be done in his/her best interests.
- Anything done or any decision made on behalf of someone who lacks capacity should be the least restrictive of his/her basic rights/freedoms.

Assessing capacity: A GP asked to give an opinion on a patient's mental capacity, should:

- Have access to the patient's records and ideally know the patient
- Seek information from friends, relatives, carers and/or the patient's independent mental capacity advocate, if one has been appointed.
- Examine the patient, and assess the type and degree of deficit
- Decide if there is an impairment of, or disturbance in, the functioning of the patient's brain or mind
- If there is a disturbance, decide if the patient is able to make the particular decision in question—in particular: Can the patient understand the information relevant to that decision, including the likely consequences of making, or not making, that decision? Can the patient retain that information? Can the patient use or weight that information as part of the process of making the decision? Can the patient communicate that decision by any means?
- Decide if assessment should be postponed while measures are taken to improve capacity
- Record all the above information.

ⓘ Even if you think a proposed action is in the patient's best interests, you must not judge the patient capable if that is not clearly the case. If in doubt, seek a second opinion.

Consent: Implies willingness of a patient to undergo examination, investigation, or treatment (collectively termed "procedure" on this page). It may be expressed (i.e. specifically says yes or no/signs a consent form) or implied (i.e. complies with the procedure without ever specifically agreeing to it—use with care). For consent to be valid patients:

- Must be competent to make the decision
- Have received sufficient information to take it; and,
- Not be acting under duress.

Information to include:
- Details of diagnosis and prognosis (including uncertainties)
- Management options—including the option not to treat and other options that you cannot offer—and for each option an estimation of likely risks, benefits and probability of success
- Reasons why you want to perform the procedure/ give the treatment proposed
- Nature, purpose and side effects (common and serious) of proposed procedure or treatment
- Whether part of a research programme or outside usual procedure
- Reminder that patients have a right to seek a second opinion and/or can change their minds about a decision at any time.
- Details of follow up in order to monitor progress or side effects.

🚺 Document if a patient does not want to be fully informed before consenting.

Mentally incapacitated adults: The Mental Capacity Act (2005), and equivalents in Scotland and Northern Ireland, enables patients' advocates (usually friends, relatives or carers) or suitable professionals (e.g. doctors, social workers), to act in patients' best interests on their behalf. This includes provision of medical care. Before acting:
- Take all factors affecting the decision into consideration
- Involve the patient with the decision making as far as possible
- Take the patient's previous known wishes into consideration, and
- Consult everyone else involved with the patient's care/welfare.

In situations in which there is disagreement about the patient's best interests, the decision can be referred to the Court of Protection

Children (<16y): A competent child is able to understand the nature, purpose and possible consequences of a proposed procedure, as well as the consequences of not undergoing that procedure. This is termed "*Gillick competence*" after the court case in which the principle was established (Gillick v West Norfolk and Wisbech AHA [1986] AC 122).

A competent child may consent to treatment . However, if treatment is refused, a parent or court may authorize procedures in the child's best interests*. Where a child is not judged competent, *only* a person with parental responsibility may authorize / refuse investigations or treatment. If in doubt, seek legal advice.

*In Scotland, parents do not have this power to overrule a competent child's decision.

Emergencies: When consent cannot be obtained, you may provide medical treatment, provided it is limited to what is immediately necessary to save life or avoid significant deterioration in the patient's health. Respect the terms of any advance statement/living will you are aware of.

Euthanasia

The word Euthanasia originates from the Greek 'eu' meaning 'good' and 'thanatos' meaning 'death'. It usually means a deliberate intervention undertaken with the express intention of ending a life so as to relieve intractable suffering, performed at the person (who dies) request or with their consent. However, some people define euthanasia to include both voluntary and involuntary termination of life.

Involuntary euthanasia: Killing of a person who has not explicitly requested aid in dying. This is most often done to patients who are in a persistent vegetative state and will probably never recover consciousness. It is not a decision a GP would ever have to make and is beyond the scope of this text.

Passive euthanasia: Hastening the death of a person by altering some form of support and letting nature take its course. Examples include the following:
- Turning off life support equipment for patients who are 'brain dead'
- Withdrawing medical procedures or treatments
- Stopping food and/or water
- Not delivering cardiopulmonary resuscitation if the patient has a cardiac or respiratory arrest
- The 'dual' or 'double' effect in which patients are given large doses of opioid analgesics to remove pain, at the cost of respiratory depression and hastening of death.

In most societies 'passive euthanasia' is acceptable for very elderly or frail patients or those with terminal illness, so that a death which was approaching comes sooner—though it is advisable to discuss any measures which may hasten death with the patient (if possible) and all close family members. If in doubt consult your medical defence body.

Where there is disagreement between family/patient and medical attendants, recourse to the courts is sometimes necessary.

Active euthanasia and physician-assisted suicide:
- Active euthanasia is death of a person through a direct action, in response to a request from that person
- In physician-assisted suicide or voluntary passive euthanasia, a physician supplies information and/or the means of committing suicide (e.g. a prescription for lethal dose of sleeping pills) to a patient so that s/he can easily terminate his/her own life.

🚯 The American state of Oregon, the Netherlands, and Belgium are the only jurisdictions in the world where laws specifically permit euthanasia or assisted suicide. Oregon permits assisted suicide; the Netherlands and Belgium permit both euthanasia and assisted suicide. Both are illegal in the UK.

Reasons why patients want to end their lives:
- **Depression:** '*A permanent solution to a temporary problem.*' There is consensus that depression should never be a reason for euthanasia—treatment is a better solution

- *Excessive pain:* This is a common reason cited for euthanasia but usually reflects inadequate clinical care. Better analgesia can give patients considerable amounts of good quality life—even if overall prognosis is poor
- *Poor quality of life/loss of dignity:* the patient has a disease which severely affects quality of life and/or dignity to the point that the patient no longer wants to live that way. Alternatively, the patient may have been diagnosed with a progressive disease which will result in a decreasing quality of life/dignity and would rather die before quality of life/dignity is lost e.g. motor neuron disease, Huntington's chorea
- *Need for control:* the patient knows s/he will die in the near future and wants control over that process with suicide as an option. In a study done in Oregon looking at the first year of legalization of physician-assisted suicide, at least 6 of the 23 patients who obtained medication to end their lives, did not use it, and actually died a natural death.

The ethical debate: The subject of voluntary euthanasia is far from simple—even the most sympathetic cases raise difficult ethical questions.

Arguments for euthanasia:
- It is a matter of personal freedom—human beings have the right to decide when and how to die
- As suicide is no longer a crime in the UK, supporters of euthanasia argue that it is not only just, but also an essential part of civilisation that people can be helped to die in dignity and painfree
- Refusing to help someone when suffering intolerable pain or distress is immoral. It could even cause more injury and distress, if the suicide attempt is botched
- Euthanasia happens anyway—it is better to have it out in the open so that it can be properly regulated and carried out
- There is no difference between withdrawing life sustaining therapy and actively ending life—in fact withdrawing life sustaining therapy may be a cruel option resulting in a more prolonged and uncomfortable death.

Arguments against euthanasia:
- Some religious groups believe life is sacrosanct and only God can decide when to terminate it. They argue we suffer for a reason
- Others believe euthanasia weakens society's belief in the sanctity of life
- Voluntary euthanasia is the start of a slippery slope—allowing any system of legalized killing would lead to patients being pushed into agreeing to euthanasia, involuntary euthanasia, and killing to save money or remove the 'undesirables' from the society
- Proper palliative care makes euthanasia unnecessary and allowing euthanasia may lead to less good care for the terminally ill
- There is no sure way of controlling euthanasia.

It is beyond the scope of this text to come to any ethical conclusions or take any stance on the debate over euthanasia.

Further information:

BBC Balanced information about the euthanasia debate and links to other sites ▢ www.bbc.co.uk/religion/ethics/euthanasia

Chapter 9

Useful information and contacts for GPs

Useful information and contacts for GPs

General information
Healthtalk Online Patient experience database
🖳 www.healthtalkonline.org

National Statistics 🖳 www.statistics.gov.uk

NICE Referral guidelines for suspected cancer (2005)
🖳 www.nice.org.uk

National Electronic Library for Health 🖳 www.library.nhs.uk

Cassidy et al. *Oxford Handbook of Oncology* (2nd edition—2006) OUP
ISBN: 0198567871

Watson M. et al. *Oncology—Oxford core text* (2nd edition—2007) OUP,
ISBN: 019856757X

Bladder cancer
NICE 🖳 www.nice.org.uk
- Improving outcomes in urological cancers (2002)
- Referral guidelines for suspected cancer (2005)
- Sunitinib for the first-line treatment of advanced and/or metastatic renal cell carcinoma (2009)

Breast cancer
NHS Breast Screening: 🖳 www.cancerscreening.org.uk

NICE 🖳 www.nice.org.uk
- Improving outcomes in breast cancer (2002)
- Familial breast cancer (2006)
- Breast cancer (early and locally advanced): diagnosis and treatment (2009)
- Breast cancer (advanced): diagnosis and treatment (2009)

Clinical Evidence 🖳 www.clinicalevidence.com
- *Stebbing et al* Breast cancer (metastatic) (2006)
- *Rodger et al* Breast cancer (non-metastatic) (2005)

Cancer Research UK Breast cancer survival statistics 🖳
www.cancerresearchuk.org/cancerstats

Cochrane *Badger et al* Physical therapies for reducing and controlling lymphoedema of the limb (2004)

Adjuvant online—decision making tool for professionals. assessing risks and benefits of additional therapy after surgery
🖳 www.adjuvantonline.com

Cancer
Cancer Research UK 🖳 www.cancerresearchuk.org

NICE Referral guidelines for suspected cancer (2005)
🖳 www.nice.org.uk

Cancer screening

National Electronic Library for Screening
⌨ www.library.nhs.uk/screening

NHS Cancer Screening Programmes
⌨ www.cancerscreening.nhs.uk

NICE Liquid based cytology for cervical screening (2003)
⌨ www.nice.org.uk

Cervical cancer

NICE Liquid based cytology for cervical screening (2003)
⌨ www.nice.org.uk

SIGN management of cervical cancer (2008) ⌨ www.sign.ac.uk

Colorectal cancer

NICE Referral guidelines for suspected cancer (2005)
⌨ www.nice.org.uk

NHS Bowel Cancer Screening Programme
⌨ www.cancerscreening.nhs.uk

SIGN Management of colorectal cancer (2007) ⌨ www.sign.ac.uk

British Society of Gastroenterology Summary of recommendations for colorectal cancer screening and surveillance in high risk groups (2002) ⌨ www.bsg.org.uk

Complementary medicine

Bandolier ⌨ www.jr2.ox.ac.uk/bandolier/booth/booths/altmed.html

Consent and decisions

GMC ⌨ www.gmc-uk.org
• Consent: patients and doctors making decisions together (2008)
• 0–18 years: guidance for all doctors (2007)

Office of the Public Guardian Making Decisions: A guide for people who work in health and social care (2007)

⌨ www.publicguardian.gov.uk

Disability and benefits

Citizens Advice Bureau ⌨ www.adviceguide.org.uk

Department of Work and Pensions. Statement of Fitness for Work: A guide for general Practitioners and other doctors
⌨ www.dwp.gov.uk/docs/fitnote-gp-guide.pdf

Direct.gov ⌨ www.direct.gov.uk/disability

Jobcentre Plus ⌨ www.jobcentreplus.gov.uk

Driving

DVLA At a glance guide to the current medical standards of fitness to drive for medical practitioners available from ⌨ www.dvla.gov.uk

Medical advisers from the DVLA can advise on difficult issues—contact: Drivers Medical Unit, DVLA, Swansea SA99 1TU or ☎ 01792 761119

217

Drugs and appliances

BNF ⌨ www.bnf.org

BNF for children 🖥 www.bnfc.org

Medicines and Healthcare products Regulatory Agency
🖥 www.mhra.gov.uk

Obtaining steroid cards:
- England and Wales: Department of Health ☎ 08701 555 455
- Scotland: Banner Business Supplies: ☎ 01506 448 440

National Prescribing Centre (NPC) *A guide to good practice in the management of controlled drugs in primary care* (England) (2007)
🖥 www.npc.co.uk

Department of Health 🖥 www.dh.gov.uk/controlleddrugs

Home Office ☎ 020 7035 4848 🖥 www.drugs.gov.uk/drugs-laws/licensing/personal

Drugs and Therapeutics Bulletin Prescribing unlicensed drugs or using drugs for unlicensed applications (1992) **30** p. 97–9

European Journal of Anaesthesiology Cohen P. Off-label use of pre-scription drugs: legal, clinical and policy considerations (1997)**14**, p. 231–50

Association of Palliative Medicine and Pain Society The use of drugs beyond licence in palliaitive care and pain management (2002)

Twycross et al *Palliative Care Formulary 2.* (2002—2ⁿᵈ edition) Radcliffe Medical Press ISBN: 1857755111

Endometrial cancer
SIGN Investigation of postmenopausal bleeding (2009)
🖥 www.sign.ac.uk

Euthanasia
BBC Balanced information about the euthanasia debate and links to other sites 🖥 www.bbc.co.uk/religion/ethics/euthanasia

GP contract
NHS Employers Primary Care Contracting 🖥 www.nhsemployers.org

Department of Health The GMS Contract. 🖥 www.dh.gov.uk

BMA The GMS contract and quality and outcomes framework
🖥 www.bma.org.uk

Head and neck cancer
SIGN Diagnosis and management of head and neck cancer (2006)
🖥 www.sign.ac.uk

Lung cancer
NICE Lung cancer: diagnosis and treatment (2005) 🖥 www.nice.org.uk

Occupational injury and disease
RIDDOR Incident contact center ☎ 0845 300 99 23
🖥 www.riddor.gov.uk

Health and Safety Executive ☎ 0845 345 0055 🖳 www.hse.gov.uk

Jobcentre plus 🖳 www.jobcentreplus.gov.uk

Occupational and Environmental Diseases Association
🖳 www.oeda.demon.co.uk

Veterans Agency ☎ 0800 169 22 77 🖳 www.veterans-uk.info

Oesophageal and gastric cancer
SIGN Management of oesophageal and gastric cancer (2006)
🖳 www.sign.ac.uk

Ovarian cancer
NICE Referral guidelines for suspected cancer (2005)
🖳 www.nice.org.uk

SIGN Epithelial ovarian cancer (2007) 🖳 www.sign.ac.uk

Cancer Research UK Ovarian cancer statistics 🖳
www.cancerresearchuk.org/cancerstats

Clayton, Monga & Baker *Gynaecology by Ten Teachers* Hodder Arnold
(2006) ISBN: 0340816627

Palliative care
Gold Standards Framework ☎ 01922 604666 🖳
www.goldstandardsframework.nhs.uk

NICE Improving supportive and palliative care for adults with cancer
(2004) 🖳 www.nice.org.uk

Hospice information ☎ 020 7520 8222
🖳 www.hospiceinformation.info

Watson, O'Reilly & Simon *Oxford GP Library: Pain and Palliation* (In Press)

Watson et al. *Oxford Handbook of Palliative Care* (2005) Oxford
University Press ISBN: 0198508972

Woodruff and Doyle *The IAHPC Manual of Palliative Care* (2004—2nd
Edition) IAHPC Press, Houston, Texas ISBN 0-9758525-1-5
🖳 www.hospicecare.com/manual/IAHPCmanual.htm

European Journal of Palliative Care Campbell C *Controlling malignant
ascites* (2001) **8** (5) p.187–191

Palliative Medicine Stephenson & Gilbert *The development of clinical
guidelines on paracentesis for ascites related to malignancy* (2002) **16**(3)
p. 213-8.

SIGN Management of pain in adults with cancer (2008)
🖳 www.sign.ac.uk

Pressure sores
NICE Pressure ulcer management (2005) 🖳 www.nice.org.uk

Prostate disease
NICE 🖳 www.nice.org.uk
- Improving outcomes in urological cancers (2002)
- Referral guidelines for suspected cancer (2005)

Cancer research UK 🖳 www.cancerresearchuk.org

National screening 🖳 www.cancerscreening.nhs.uk

Skin cancer

British Association of Dermatologists 🖳 www.bad.org.uk
- Guidelines for the management of BCC (2008)
- Guidelines for management of Bowen's disease (2006)
- Multiprofessional guidelines for the management of the patient with primary cutaneous squamous cell carcinoma (2009)
- UK guidelines for the management of cutaneous melanoma (2002)

NICE Improving outcomes for people with skin tumours including melanoma: The Manual (2006) 🖳 www.nice.org.uk

SIGN Diagnosis and management of head and neck cancer (2006) 🖳 www.sign.ac.uk

Vulval cancer

RCOG Management of vulval cancer (2006) 🖳 www.rcog.org.uk

Information and contacts for patients, relatives and carers

General information
Healthtalk Online patient experience database
🖳 www.healthtalkonline.org

Patient UK Patient information on a range of topics
🖳 www.patient.co.uk

Benefits
Benefit fraud line ☎ 0800 85 44 40

Citizens Advice Bureau 🖳 www.adviceguide.org.uk

Department of Work and Pensions 🖳 www.dwp.gov.uk
☎ *Benefits Enquiry Line*—0800 882200; 0800 243355 (minicom facility);
0800 441144 (for help with form completion).

Government information and services 🖳 www.direct.gov.uk

HM Revenue and Customs 🖳 www.hmrc.gov.uk

Jobcentre Plus 🖳 www.jobcentreplus.gov.uk

Pension service 🖳 www.thepensionservice.gov.uk

Pensions Advisory Service (TPA) ☎ 0845 601 2923
🖳 www.pensionsadvisoryservice.org.uk

Veterans Agency ☎ 0800 169 22 77 🖳 www.veterans-uk.info

Brain tumours
Brain Tumour UK ☎ 0845 4500 386 🖳 www.braintumouruk.org.uk

Brain and spine foundation ☎ 0808 808 1000
🖳 www.brainandspine.org.uk

Breast cancer
Cancer screening UK 🖳 www.cancerscreening.org.uk
● Breast Screening—the Facts
● Over 70? You are still entitled to breast screening

Breakthrough breast cancer 🖳 www.breakthrough.org.uk

Breast Cancer Care ☎ 0808 800 6000 🖳
www.breastcancercare.org.uk

Breast Cancer Campaign 🖳 www.bcc-uk.org

Against Breast Cancer 🖳 www.aabc.org.uk

Cancer
Macmillan Cancer Support ☎ 0808 808 0000
🖳 www.macmillan.org.uk

CancerHelp UK ☎ 0808 800 4040 🖳 www.cancerhelp.org.uk

Carers

NHS Carers Direct ☎ 0808 802 0202 ▢ www.nhs.uk/carersdirect

Carers UK ☎ 0808 808 7777 ▢ www.carersuk.org

Counsel and Care ☎ 0845 300 7585 ▢ www.counselandcare.org.uk

Princess Royal Trust for Carers ☎ 0844 800 4361
▢ www.carers.org

Disability and carers service ▢ www.direct.gov.uk/carers or
www.direct.gov.uk/disability

Caring with Confidence. ▢ www.caringwithconfidence.net

Cervical cancer

Cervical Screening—the Facts ▢ www.cancerscreening.nhs.uk

Chemotherapy

Chemocare ▢ www.chemocare.com

Colorectal cancer

Colostomy Association ☎ 0800 328 4257
▢ www.colostomyassociation.org.uk

Bowel cancer screening—the Facts ▢ www.cancerscreening.org.uk

Elderly

Age UK ☎ 0800 169 65 65 ▢ www.ageuk.org.uk

Head and neck cancer

Mouth cancer foundation ▢ www.rdoc.org.uk

ENT UK ▢ www.entuk.org

Leukaemia

Leukaemia Care ☎ 0800 169 6680 ▢ www.leukaemiacare.org

Leukaemia Society ▢ www.leukaemiasociety.org

Leukaemia and Lymphoma Research ▢ www.llresearch.org.uk

Children with Leukaemia ☎ 020 7404 0808
▢ www.leukaemia.org.uk

CLIC and Sargent ☎ 0800 197 0068 ▢ www.clicsargent.org.uk

Lung cancer

The Roy Castle Lung Cancer Foundation ▢ www.roycastle.org

Lung cancer resources directory ▢ www.cancerindex.org

British Lung foundation ☎ 08458 50 50 20 ▢ www.lunguk.org

Lymphoedema

Lymphoedema support network ☎ 020 7351 4480 ▢
www.lymphoedema.org/lsn

UKLymph.com On-line support network ▢ www.uklymph.com

Skin Care Campaign ▢ www.skincarecampaign.org

Lymphoma
Lymphoma Association ☎ 0808 808 5555 ⌨ www.lymphomas.org.uk

Mouth cancer—see oral cancer

Neuroblastoma
Neuroblastoma society ☎ 020 8940 4353 ⌨ www.nsoc.co.uk

Oesophageal cancer
Oesophageal patients' association ☎ 021 704 9860
⌨ www.opa.org.uk

Oral cancer
Mouth cancer foundation ⌨ www.rdoc.org.uk

ENT UK Information on Head and Neck Cancer ⌨ www.entuk.org

Ovarian cancer
Ovacome ☎ 0845 371 0554 ⌨ www.ovacome.org.uk

Pituitary disease
The Pituitary Foundation ☎ 0845 450 0375 ⌨ www.pituitary.org.uk

Prostate cancer
National screening ⌨ www.cancerscreening.nhs.uk

Prostate cancer charity ☎ 0800 074 8383
⌨ www.prostate-cancer.org.uk

Prostate cancer support association ☎ 0845 601 0766
⌨ www.prostatecancersupport.co.uk

Retinoblastoma
Childhood eye cancer trust (CHECT) ☎ 020 7377 5578
⌨ www.chect.org.uk

Sarcoma
Sarcoma UK ⌨ www.sarcoma-uk.org

Skin cancer
Cancer Research UK Sun Smart Campaign
⌨ www.cancerresearchuk.org/SunSmart

British Association of Dermatologists ⌨ www.bad.org.uk

Thyroid cancer
British Thyroid Foundation ⌨ www.btf-thyroid.org

Index

A

abdominal distension, children 50

abdominal masses 41, 43, 136
children 50, 158, 159

abdominal pain 40, 48
management 166

accelerated chronic myeloid leukaemia 140

achievement payments 9

aciclovir, for cold sores 169

acoustic neuromas 145

acral lentiginous melanoma 148

active euthanasia 212

activities of daily living, Karnofsky score 12, 13

acute leukaemia
bone marrow investigation 135
differential diagnosis 132
information sources for patients, relatives, and carers 223
initial management 133
investigation 132
presentation 132
prognosis 134
prognostic factors 135
sources of information and support 135
specialist management 134
treatment phases 134

acute lymphoblastic leukaemia (ALL) 132
see also acute leukaemia

acute myeloid leukaemia (AML) 132
see also acute leukaemia

adaptations 197

additional services 8

adenoid cystic carcinoma 152

adenomatous polyps 128

adjuvant treatment 58
chemotherapy 65
radiotherapy 62

adrenal cortex tumours 156

adrenaline, for bleeding wounds 85, 179

Adriamycin® (doxorubicin) 67

adult cancers
incidence 2
survival rates 6

age at diagnosis, relationship to survival rates 6

age of death 4

alarm symptoms
bone cancer/sarcoma 48
childhood cancer 50–1
haematological malignancies 48–9
head and neck 38–9
lower GI tract 41
lung cancer 46
mouth 40
skin cancer 46–7
upper GI tract 40–1
urological 44–5
women's cancers 42–3

alarm systems 197

alcohol-induced pain 48

alcohol intake 16
and breast cancer risk 98
and colorectal cancer risk 128

Alimta® (pemetrexed) 70

alpha-feto-protein (α FP) 55
in liver cancer 127
in ovarian cancers 108

amelanotic melanoma 148

amitriptyline, for excessive salivation 169

amyloidosis, in myeloma 142

anaemia 48, 171

anal cancer 130

analgesia 164
drugs for use in syringe drivers 185
morphine equivalent conversions 165
opioid toxicity 165
palliative radiotherapy 62
palliative surgery 61
specific types of pain 166
mouth pain 169
wounds 179
troubleshooting 165
use of morphine 167
WHO analgesics ladder 165

anaplastic large cell lymphoma 137
see also non-Hodgkin's lymphoma (NHL)

anastrozole (Arimidex®) 73, 100

aniridia 159

Ann Arbor staging of lymphoma 139

anterior pituitary gland tumours 156

anti-androgens 73
in prostate cancer 116–17

antibiotics
combination with analgesics 164
in neutropaenic sepsis 90

anticoagulation 86

anticonvulsants, combination with analgesics 164

antidepressants, combination with analgesics 164

anti-emetic ladder 172

anti-emetics
with morphine 167
in palliative care 172–3

anti-oestrogens 73

antispasmodics 164

anxiety
as cause of vomiting 173
due to breast cancer screening 24
terminal 182

aperients 175

Arimidex® (anastrozole) 73, 100

Armed Forces Compensation Scheme (AFCS) 189

asbestos exposure 16, 46
compensation for industrial lung disease 199
notification 198

ascites, management 174
paracentesis 76

ascorbic acid, for coated tongue 169

aspiration payments 9

aspirin, for diarrhoea 175

assessment of tumours 54

astrocytomas 145

ataxia telangiectasia 136

atropine, for excessive salivation 169

Attendance Allowance (AA) 194, 200

Avastin® (bevacizumab) 72

225

Q

R